Facilitating
Classroom Listening

Facilitating Classroom Listening

Frederick S. Berg, Ph.D.

Utah State University
Department of Communicative Disorders
College of Education
Logan, Utah

A Handbook for Teachers of
Normal and Hard of Hearing Students

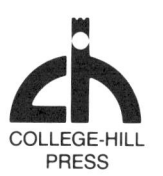

COLLEGE-HILL
PRESS

A College-Hill Publication

Little, Brown and Company
Boston/Toronto/San Diego

College-Hill Press,
A Division of
Little, Brown and Company (Inc.)
34 Beacon Street
Boston, Massachusetts 02108

© 1987 by Little, Brown and Company (Inc.)

All rights, including that of translation, reserved. No part of this publication may be reproduced, stored in a retrieval system, or transmitted in any form or by any means, electronic, mechanical, recording, or otherwise, without the prior written permission of the publisher.

Library of Congress Cataloging in Publication Data
Main entry under title:

  Berg, Frederick S.
    Facilitating Classroom Listening.

    Bibliography: p. 201
    Includes index.
    1. Hearing impaired children—Education.
    2. Listening. 3. Classroom environment. 4. Noise pollution. 5. Hearing aids. I. Title.
    HV2483.B48   1987   371.91′2   86–14760
    ISBN 0-316-09144-8

ISBN 0-316-09144-8

Printed in the United States of America

CONTENTS

Preface		v
Chapter 1.	*Basic Considerations*	1
Chapter 2.	*Hearing Considerations*	17
Chapter 3.	*Speech Considerations*	39
Chapter 4.	*Listening Considerations*	63
Chapter 5.	*Room Acoustics*	89
Chapter 6.	*Hearing Aids*	117
Chapter 7.	*FM Equipment*	155
Glossary		191
References		201
Subject Index		207

PREFACE

Excessive noise and reverberation in classrooms and high prevalence of hearing loss are common among students in the elementary and secondary schools of the nation. These problems are major contributors to listening and learning difficulties experienced by school children. Poor classroom acoustics cause even normal students to have listening difficulty. Students with hearing loss experience more severe listening difficulty. Learning and education are correspondingly adversely affected.

This book focuses on how to minimize hearing loss, noise, and reverberation, and how to alleviate the resulting adverse listening and educational effects. It is the main product of a current study supported by the U. S. Department of Education, involving many universities and school districts, and entitled Project Listening in Urban and Rural Noise (LURN). It is a text or major reference for preservice and inservice training in elementary, secondary, and special education, and in audiology, education of the hearing impaired, and speech-language pathology.

Concepts for understanding acoustics and hearing and their effects on listening, and skills for compensating for acoustic, hearing, and listening problems, are presented in this book. In the first chapter, parameters of the problem are introduced and the rationale for teacher involvement is explained. Each of the remaining six chapters extends the discussion of the problem and builds upon previous solutions. Hearing considerations, speech considerations, listening considerations, room acoustics, hearing aids, and frequency modulation (FM) equipment are covered, in that order. In each chapter, the roles of specialists and classroom teachers are described.

The entire book can be used as a text for a course, or chapters of the book can be used as topics for study. Skills to be learned by teachers are identified throughout the book. Lecture outlines, slides, video demonstrations, and further equipment and material information can be obtained by writing the author.

In Chapter 1, "Basic Considerations," the listening problem and classroom teacher roles are introduced. The involvement of audiologists, educators of the hearing impaired, and speech-language pathologists in classroom listening management is described. A discussion of individualized educational programs (IEPs) is included in an appendix to this chapter.

In Chapter 2, "Hearing Considerations," the role of hearing is explained, the hearing mechanism described, hearing loss discussed, hearing conservation detailed, and behavioral symptoms of hearing impairment listed.

In Chapter 3, "Speech Considerations," the speech mechanism is described, the effects of hearing loss on speech explained, the sounds of speech detailed, speech screening and parent guidance discussed, an electronic speech aid introduced, and speech programs outlined.

In the fourth chapter, "Listening Considerations," definitions and processes of listening are reviewed, listening development explained, the use of the audiometer and audiograms described, understanding speech discussed, hearing screening detailed, simulating hearing loss covered, and the five sound test introduced. A comprehensive listening test is explained, and specific listening tasks illustrated.

In Chapter 5, "Room Acoustics," the definitions and processes pertaining to this topic are developed, classroom listening data reviewed, measurement and calculation explained, procedures for reducing reverberation and noise detailed, and an acoustical control plan for a school outlined.

In Chapter 6, "Hearing Aids," what a hearing aid does is explained, types of aids are described, candidates for aids specified, features of behind-the-ear (BTE) and in-the-ear (ITE) aids and earmolds detailed, and basic components of aids discussed. A hearing aid management program is outlined, with focus on daily checking and servicing of specific problem areas.

The last chapter (7) is entitled "FM Equipment." Frequency modulation (FM) radio transmission is explained, candidates for sound field FM equipment and personal FM equipment are described, FM components and accessories detailed, the operation of one brand of personal FM equipment prescribed, evaluation and maintenance steps outlined, and evaluation materials included.

Several means have been used to interest classroom teachers as well as communicative disorders specialists in this book. First, case studies introduce chapter discussions. Second, technical areas are discussed with common terminology and clarified with many illustrations. Third, text material is free of author citations. Fourth, further readings appear at the ends of chapters. Fifth, serious students can find technical explanations in chapter appendices. Sixth, a glossary of terms, a shortened list of references, and a subject index appear at the end of the book.

Additional means have been used to interest audiologists, educators of the hearing impaired, and speech-language pathologists in the book. First, updates on related educational audiology studies are included. Second, state-of-the-art equipment and technologies are described. Third, ideas for working with classroom teachers are suggested. Fourth, sources of further specialized information are included.

Still additional means have been made to interest parents of school children in this book. First, information on room acoustics can be generalized from the school to the home. Second, hearing loss and its secondary consequences are clarified. Third, parental roles and tasks in solving problems are implied in many discussions. Fourth, parents will discover new ways for elementary, secondary, and special education teachers to help their children listen and learn more effectively.

Numerous individuals have assisted me with the preparation of this book: James C. Blair, James S. Cangelosi, Dee R. Child, Lynette Crookston, Kathleen C. Drebin, Diane Heaps, Thomas S. Johnson, Ruth Struyk, and Steven H. Viehweg of Utah State University; Steven P. Bornstein of Columbia University; Wendy D. Hanks of University of Nevada-Reno; Robert M. Traynor of Colorado State University; Harold Utty of the University of Central Florida; and Diane Williams of San Diego State University. Dr. Daniel Ling of the University of Western Ontario has read the entire manuscript. Anna Congdon provided exceptional editing. College-Hill Press personnel have helped, including Sadanand Singh, Marie Linvill, Ted Logan, Linda Nevin, Linda Wooten, who assisted with artwork, and Susan Altman, who ably managed the editorial production. My family has offered their support.

The following persons, publishers, copyright holders, organizations, and agencies have kindly given permission to use figures, quoted materials, tables, and other materials: Activar, Jerry Agnew, Amera, American Otological Society, Archives of Otolaryngology, Audio Enhancement, Audiotone, Alexander Graham Bell Association for the Deaf, American Speech-Language-Hearing Association, Edna Berg, Bernafon, James Blair, Arthur Boothroyd, Columbia Dispatch, Comtek, Communication Skill Builders, Halowell Davis, Dover, Eckel, Endeco Medical, Norman Erber, Frye Electronics, Victor Goodhill, Grune & Stratton, Hal-Hen, Harper and Row, Hearing Aid Journal, Hearing Instruments, Terese Finitzo-Hieber, Holt, Rinehart & Winston, Industrial Acoustics, James Jerger, Daniel Johnson, Jerry Jones, Krames Communications, Peter Ladefoged, Larson-Davis, Stanton Leggett, G. A. Levow, Samuel Lybarger, Maico, McGraw-Hill, Caroline Musket, Anna Nabelek, Oticon, Phillips, Phonic Ear, Prentice-Hall, Pro-Ed, Qualitone, Stephen Quigley, Rastronics, Rion, Mark Ross, Lewis Sarff, Scientific American, Charlann Simon, Sonotone, Wayne Staab, Tandy, Telex, Thieme-Stratton, Unitron, University of Chicago, Utah State University, Steven Viehweg, Welsh-Allen, Joel Wernick, Widex, John Wiley & Sons, World Book, and Zenetron.

Chapter 1

Basic Considerations

LISTENING PROBLEMS IN THE SCHOOLS

Hearing Loss

In the United States nearly 8 million of the 39 million school children may have varying degrees of hearing loss in one or both ears (Fig. 1-1). The degree of hearing loss need only be minimal to cause educational deficit. By the time many hard of hearing children finish elementary school, they are two or more years behind academically. Relatively more hard of hearing students than normal hearing students do not complete high school.

Secondary Consequences

The hard of hearing child presents a bewildering complexity of problems to consider. These problems encompass listening, speech, language, cognition and academics, emotions and social relations, parental and societal reactions, and vocational performance. The most frequent and most basic secondary consequence of hearing loss is listening deficit. A simple test for experiencing just a minimal hearing loss is to press the tabs in front of your ears tightly into the ear canals. Then, try listening to someone talk or try carrying on a conversation with someone. Even this degree of loss interferes seriously with listening. A hearing loss in one ear also interferes with listening and learning in school.

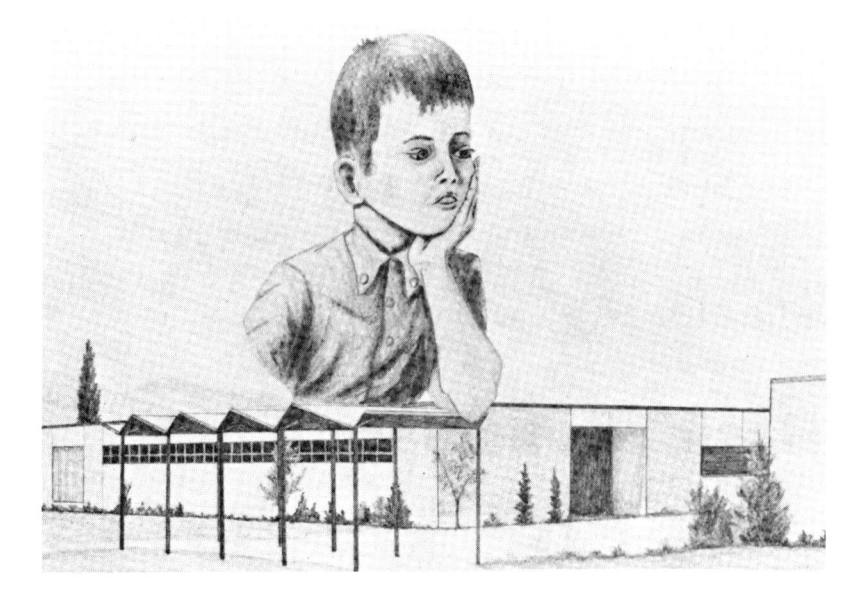

Figure 1-1. The neglected and forgotten hard of hearing child. From Berg, F. (1971). *Breakthrough for the hard of hearing child* (p. 26). Smithfield, UT: Ear Publication. Reprinted by permission.

Classroom Acoustics

Hard of hearing children in both regular and special classrooms are in need of classroom support in listening. Unfortunately, rather than providing listening help, the classroom itself further compounds the listening problem of hard of hearing children. The typical classroom is noisy and reverberant, making it difficult for even normal hearing students to hear all of what the teacher is saying. Hard of hearing children are even more susceptible to listening breakdown than normal hearing children under the same conditions of poor classroom acoustics. The fact that a hard of hearing child may be wearing a hearing aid does not help much when noise and reverberation are present. The aid amplifies unwanted sounds as well as wanted sounds. The teacher's voice often tires just trying to talk above the noise level.

Auditory Processing Difficulty

In addition to the hard of hearing, many other children have listening problems. Their problem is not with detecting the presence of sound but with processing in their brains the sound they do hear. Children with central auditory processing problems may respond inconsistently to directions, or have short attention spans, or show extreme distractibility. In a noisy or reverberant classroom, auditory processing difficulty is accentuated.

Role of Listening in School

Listening is particularly important to children during their early language learning years. Often the hearing loss or auditory processing problem is not discovered until age 5, and the child begins kindergarten with a language problem that makes listening even more difficult. To listen effectively is crucial to school learning because students spend 45 percent of school time listening and 30 percent speaking, but only 16 percent reading and 9 percent writing.

PERSONNEL NEEDED

Audiologists

American education has not yet come to grips with overcoming or alleviating the listening problems of hard of hearing children. Audiologists have responsibility for school children with hearing loss, but they spend little time in school classrooms. There is a need for 8000 school audiologists, but only 400 audiologists are employed by the schools (Fig. 1–2). The relatively few audiologists working in the schools perceive their job task to be primarily identification and diagnosis of children with hearing loss rather than classroom management of hard of hearing students. Educational audiologists take responsibility for hearing aids that are referred to them, but they spend little time training teachers to manage these aids. They give even less time to classroom acoustics and classroom amplification equipment.

Speech-Language Pathologists

Thousands of speech-language pathologists assist in identifying children with hearing loss in the schools, but they also do not perceive their job task to include the management of hard of hearing children. Their caseloads tend to be made up of children with speech and language disorders unrelated to hearing loss. The relatively few speech-language pathologists who do assist hard of hearing children limit their efforts to communication training conducted outside of classrooms. Speech-language pathologists rate their competence in providing hearing aid or classroom amplification services to be very low.

4 Facilitating Classroom Listening

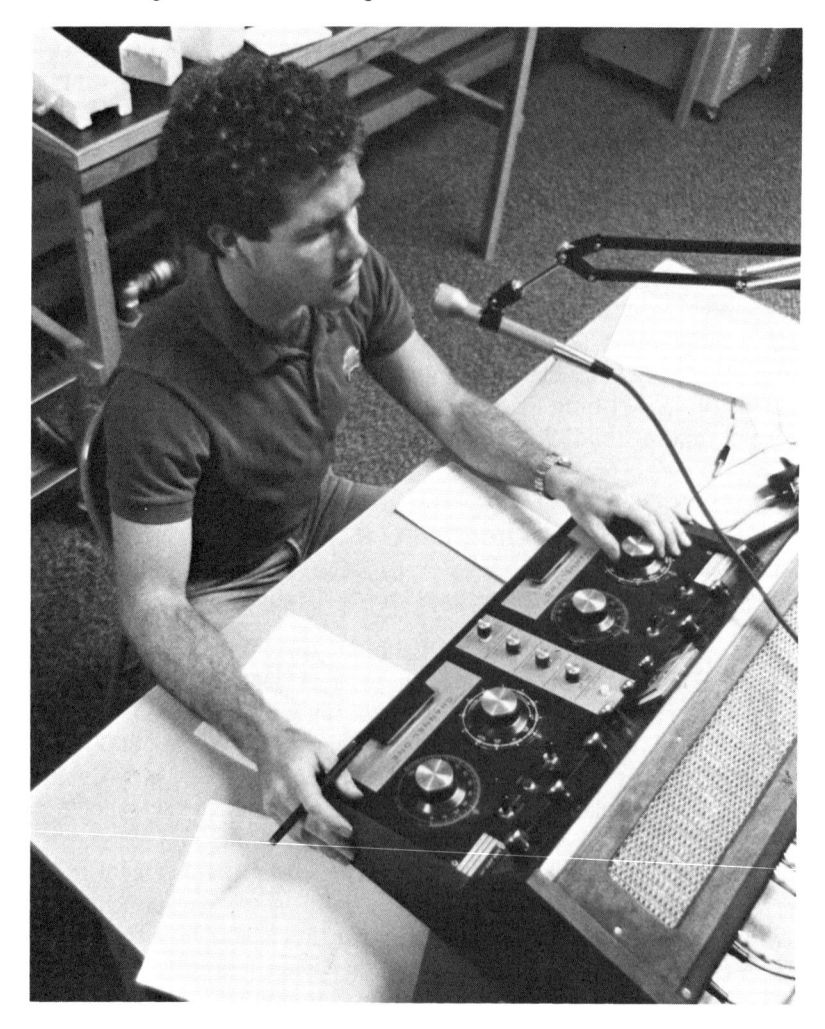

Figure 1-2. An audiologist using an audiometer to conduct hearing tests. From Berg, F. (1983). *Listening in classrooms: Handbook for hard-of-hearing students* (p. 1). Logan, UT: Utah State University. Reprinted by permission.

Teachers of the Hearing Impaired

Historically, teachers of the deaf have directly taught hearing impaired (deaf and hard of hearing) children and youth, in contrast to the lack of educational involvement of audiologists and speech-language pathologists. This training is conducted mainly in special schools and classes and often uses methods developed for teaching the deaf rather than the hard of hearing. With the passage of the All Handicapped

Children's Act in 1974, more teachers of the deaf now tutor hearing impaired children who are mainstreamed into regular classrooms. However, the hearing management skills of the majority of teachers of the deaf are minimal because of lack of preservice course work in using residual hearing. Many mainstream or itinerant teachers of the deaf have had little experience with classroom acoustics, hearing aids, or classroom amplification equipment, which severely restricts their ability to serve the hard of hearing. In addition, most of these professionals have had limited experience with audiograms and tympanograms, which if interpreted correctly could help both hard of hearing and near deaf children.

Regular and Special Educators

Generally, no one in the schools deals with the management of residual hearing or listening problems of hard of hearing children. Since neither the audiologist, the speech-language pathologist, nor the teacher of the deaf is inclined or prepared to assist hard of hearing children to listen in school classrooms, teachers of elementary, secondary, and special education students will have to provide this assistance if it is to be given. Traditionally, however, career educators have not enrolled in course work related to hearing loss in their programs of professional preparation. Therefore, career educators are not now prepared to assist with the listening problems of the great numbers of children in their own classrooms. For the benefit of all children with hearing loss or auditory processing problems, and normal hearing children as well, there is need to provide special training in listening management to teachers of elementary, secondary, and special education classrooms.

CLASSROOM TEACHER ROLES

The more than one million elementary, secondary, and special education teachers in the United States have responsibility to educate all children enrolled in their classrooms, including youngsters with hearing problems (Fig. 1–3). Before appropriate education can be provided, however, there is need to identify and seek help for pathologic ear conditions, hearing loss, and resultant speech and listening deficits among their students. Professional preparation programs have already oriented teachers to language, academic, emotional, social, and parental problems that exist among children and to Individualized Educational Plans and Programs (IEPs) for handicapped students. Teachers also need to be able to identify noise and reverberation problems of their classrooms

6 Facilitating Classroom Listening

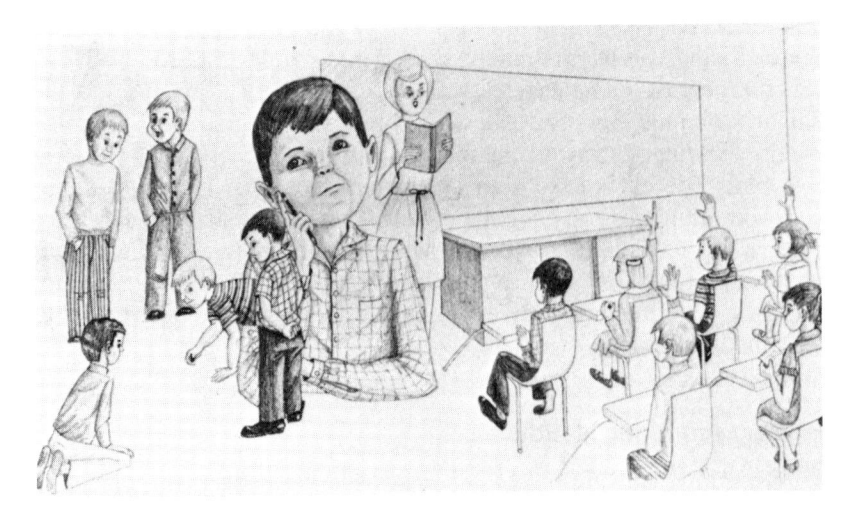

Figure 1.3. A classroom teacher and a neglected hard of hearing child. From Berg, F. (1971). *Breakthrough for the hard of hearing child* (p. 32). Smithfield, UT: Ear Publication. Reprinted by permission.

that prevent optimal listening and know of steps to alleviate these inhibitors to learning. Finally, teachers need to understand when children need hearing aids and FM systems and how to operate and maintain individual and classroom amplification equipment.

Hearing Problems

Temporary and permanent hearing loss is ordinarily due to various types of pathologic conditions of the ear. Each part of each ear and auditory nerve pathway of a child must be intact before the complete sound signal can reach the brain to be fully detected and comprehended. There are all degrees of hearing loss, a great many conditions causing it, and a high prevalence of hearing loss among children. In each school classroom there are also youngsters who are presumed to have minimal brain damage causing auditory processing problems. Hearing loss is typical of many children in special education classrooms. Teachers should be aware of how audiologists identify pathologic conditions of the ear and hearing problems. They should learn to recognize physical signs and behaviors that are symptomatic of hearing loss and auditory processing problems among children.

Speech Problems

When a child has a hearing loss in both ears, the child's speech is often defective. A speech defect interferes with speaking and is socially and emotionally undesirable. The greater the hearing loss and the earlier in life its onset, the greater the speech problem. Hearing loss may be serious enough to make it difficult for the child to learn to pronounce words and to learn to use spoken language. Reading and writing deficits accompany speech and spoken language problems. The teacher should take time to learn to recognize the sounds of speech in words and to identify when a child makes mistakes in articulating them. The teacher should also be able to assist the speech-language pathologist or teacher of the hearing impaired in the speech training of hearing impaired children.

Listening Problems

Whenever a child has any degree of hearing loss, in one or both ears, a listening problem also exists. Many children also have listening problems in the sense of having auditory processing difficulties. When a classroom is noisy or reverberant, even normal children do not listen effectively. When teachers do not talk loud enough or do not face their students when they talk, listening is more difficult. It is particularly important to young children learning language that they be able to listen very effectively. In the first years of school, it is extremely important that children hear, classroom acoustics be desirable or classroom amplification be provided, and teachers communicate effectively. The teacher can assist specialists by monitoring the progress of students in learning to listen and lipread. They can also participate in listening training.

Acoustical Problems

For classroom teachers to be heard, their voices must reach their students loudly enough and without interference. Teachers must vary the loudness of their voices to compensate for close and distant instruction. When classrooms are noisy, which is usually the case, teachers must raise their voices to be heard from any distance. When room surfaces are hard, sound reverberation exists, and the teacher's voice cannot be heard clearly. Teachers should learn of simple ways to identify and measure or calculate room noise and reverberation. They should also understand what needs to be done to rooms to bring noise and reverberation within acceptable instructional levels (Fig. 1–4).

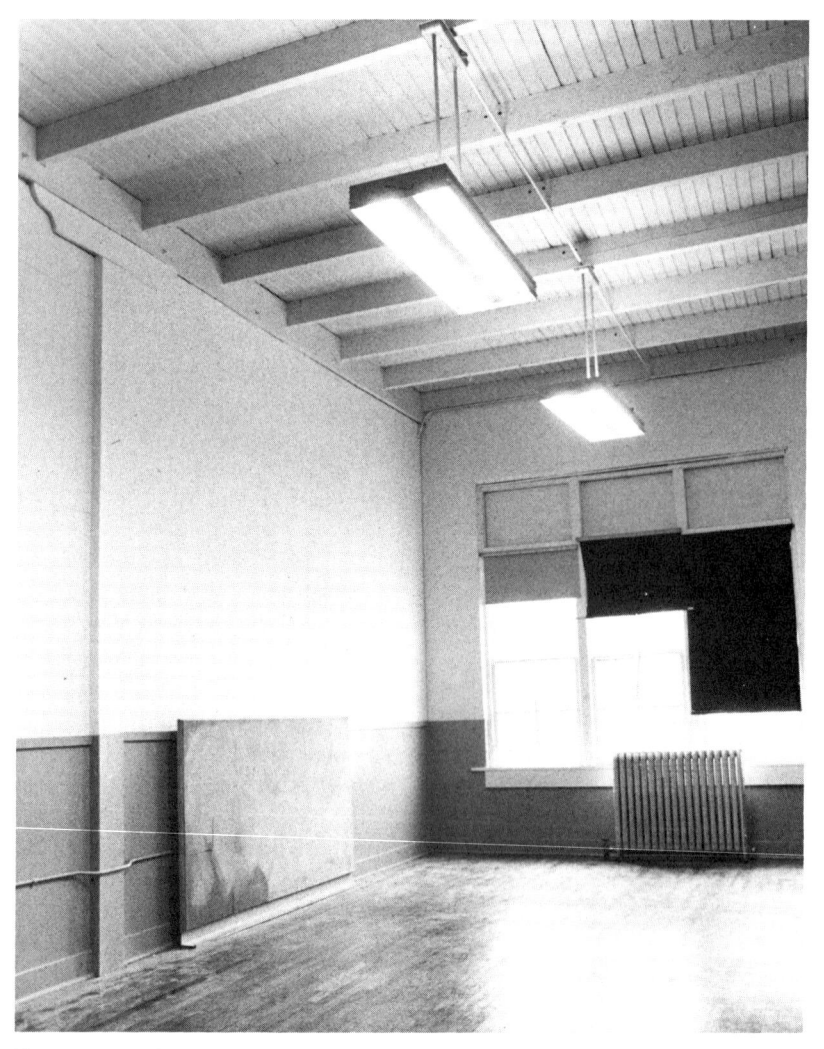

Figure 1-4. An old classroom with hard surfaces and a noisy radiator. From Berg, F., et al. (1983). *Listening in classrooms, hard of hearing* (p. 179). Logan, UT: Utah State University. Reprinted by permission.

Hearing Aids

In each class there are students who can benefit educationally from hearing aids. An appropriately selected hearing aid will amplify sound to partially compensate for the user's hearing loss. Certain nearby sounds that cannot be heard without an aid will be heard with an aid. More distant sounds will also be heard with an aid than without it. Students currently using hearing aids are those with the most serious hearing losses, although students with lesser degrees of loss can also benefit from them. Teen-age students resist wearing hearing aids that are visible to others. Many parents also resist the fitting of hearing aids on their children. Personal hearing aids are most effective in quiet classrooms that have soft surfaces. A hearing aid needs constant care to be as effective as possible. Teachers need to be as familiar as possible with the advantages and limitations of hearing aids. They also need to know how to conduct basic visual and listening checks of hearing aids and to refer problems to audiologists, and need to understand their role in an overall hearing aid management program.

FM Equipment

Unless a classroom is quiet and has soft surfaces, it should be equipped with a room amplification system to enhance the listening of all students (Fig. 1–5). The most versatile room amplification system is frequency modulation (FM) radio equipment. The teacher wears a mobile microphone and FM transmitter. Students with hearing aids wear FM radio receivers, which are coupled to their hearing aids. Students with minimal hearing loss, central auditory processing problems, or normal listening capabilities listen to the teacher with the aid of a classroom FM receiver, amplifier, and loudspeakers. FM equipment enables teachers to instruct their students from any distance without raising their voices. Noise and reverberation becomes background rather than foreground sound. Teachers should understand how to operate, evaluate, and maintain FM equipment.

SUMMARY

Hearing problems are so prevalent and room acoustics so poor in our nation's schools that elementary, secondary, and special education teachers need a special course on classroom listening. Listening problems in classrooms are experienced by children with hearing loss, youngsters with presumed minimal brain damage, and students with normal capabilities. Specialists such as audiologists, speech-language pathologists, and teachers of the hearing impaired are not meeting the classroom listening needs of school children. To combat listening problems in the classroom, a teacher needs to assume roles in the identification of hearing loss, speech deficits, listening problems, and undesirable classroom acoustics and in the management of hearing aids and mobile classroom amplification equipment.

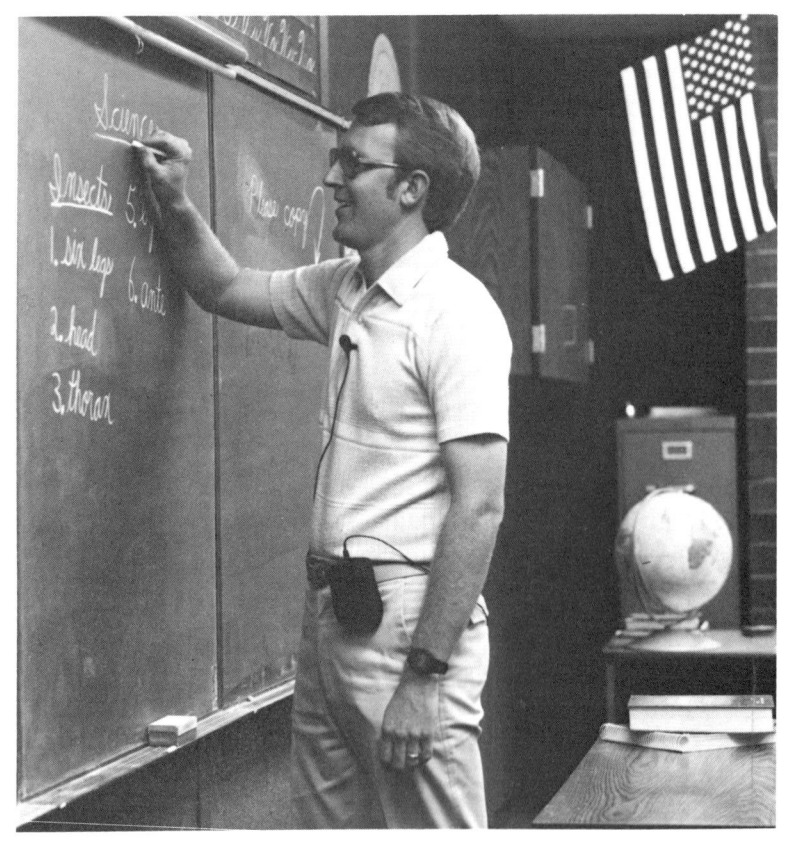

Figure 1-5. A classroom teacher using FM equipment to reach his students while his back is turned. From Omni-2000 advertisement by C. Anderson. Orem, UT: Audio Enhancement Systems. Reprinted by permission.

FURTHER READINGS

Arthur Boothroyd's *Hearing Impairments in Young Children* (Prentice-Hall, Englewood Cliffs, NJ, 1982) is a developmentally conceived parent and teacher guidebook on the management of preschool deaf and hard of hearing children. A comprehensive sourcebook on the foundations of verbal learning in hearing impaired children is Daniel and Agnes Ling's *Aural Habilitation* (Alexander Graham Bell Association for the Deaf, Washington, DC, 1978). An insightful monograph on psychosocial asects of hearing loss written by hearing impaired persons and edited by Richard Stoker and Jack Spears is *Hearing Impaired Perspectives on Living in the Mainstream* (The Volta Review, Alexander Graham Bell Association for the Deaf, Washington, DC,

1984). Jack Birch's *Hearing Impaired Children in the Mainstream* (The Council for Exceptional Children, Reston, VA, 1975) provides a broad sourcebook of hearing management ideas for the regular teacher and school administrators. A chapter on meeting state and federal guidelines of the Education of All Handicapped Children Act of 1975 (Public Law 94-142) has been written by Carol Amon in the valuable volume entitled *Auditory Disorders in School Children* (Thieme-Stratton, New York, 1981). A specialized book on how the audiologist can help the teacher, called *Educational Audiology for the Hard of Hearing Child* (Grune & Stratton, Orlando, FL, 1986), has recently been written by Frederick Berg, James Blair, Steven Viehweg, and Ann Wilson-Vlotman. Another specialized sourcebook in educational audiology, called *Hard of Hearing Children in Regular Schools* (Prentice-Hall, Englewood Cliffs, NJ, 1982), has been written by Mark Ross with assistance from Diane Brackett and Antonio Maxon. The educational neglect of the hard of hearing child is described in the booklet by Julia Davis entitled *Our Forgotten Children: Hard of Hearing Pupils in the Schools* (University of Minnesota Press, Minneapolis, 1977).

APPENDIX

Individualized Educational Program (IEP)

Public Law 94-142, the All Handicapped Children's Act, has this mandate: *All children who are handicapped and in need of special education and related services must be identified, located, evaluated, and assured a free appropriate education in the least restrictive environment.* An appropriate education for each handicapped child is to be developed with an individualized educational plan (IEP) and implemented in an individualized educational program (IEP). In the United States, IEPs are written annually for about 41,000 deaf students and 41,000 hard of hearing students. The number of IEPs written for hard of hearing students is far fewer than need to be written. The law covers hard of hearing students if they require special education, speech assistance, amplification, and related audiologic services.

According to the regulations of the law, each IEP should (1) provide an overview of the student's learning style or constraints, (2) detail the general and specific objectives for the student for the coming school year, (3) document professional services that are necessary to achieve the stated objectives, and (4) address the measures and criteria to be used to determine alternative services or placement.

To meet these objectives, a student study team prepares individualized assessments and confers collectively to complete the IEP. Regulations stipulate that team members include parents, teachers, an administrator, and the handicapped student (where appropriate). The team should be expanded to include specialists such as the educational audiologist, the speech-language pathologist, the educator of the hearing impaired, and the school psychologist. Each aspect of identification (hearing screening, speech/language screening, and academic performance), assessment (educational, psychological, speech/language/hearing), and placement of the hard of hearing student should be considered by team members (Nober, 1981).

An underlying principle of the law is to place handicapped students in the least restrictive environment. Generally, hard of hearing students receiving IEPs continue to be enrolled in regular classrooms. Mentally retarded students with hearing loss, however, are usually enrolled in special classrooms.

Elementary, secondary, and special education classroom teachers have important roles in identification and evaulation of hard of hearing students. In addition, they are very much involved in the special services that are provided students with hearing loss.

When the All Handicapped Children's Law was first interpreted, hearing screening levels for identifying hard of hearing students were set at 25 to 30 dB. This procedure resulted in failure to identify many, if not most, students with hearing loss. With hearing screening levels now tending to be set at 15 dB, the special educational needs of a much larger number of hard of hearing students are being uncovered.

Identifying Hard of Hearing Children

The problem of identifying hard of hearing children extends from the preschool years through the elementary and secondary years. The specific task is to distinguish the hard of hearing child from the normally hearing child and from the deaf child. One purpose of this recognition is simply to take a first step in providing appropriate educational services for the hard of hearing. In the past, the hard of hearing child has tended to be educated either as a normally hearing youngster or as a deaf child, without due consideration being given to the varying communication abilities of these three populations. Communicatively, the hard of hearing child is more like the normal hearing child than like the deaf child, because both use audition rather than vision as the primary mode for speech and language development and usage. However, the hard of hearing child will be neglected in both the regular class and the special class unless recognition is given to that child's unique communication problems (Berg, 1986).

The measurement of hearing contributes to the differentiation of the hard of hearing child from the normal hearing child and from the deaf child. If the child has a hearing loss for speech of 15 dB or less in the better ear, that child often can be considered a normal hearing child. If the hearing loss is 16 dB or greater, the child can be called hard of hearing, unless the loss is so great that audition is no longer the primary communicative input mode. On the average, 95 to 100 dB is a dividing line between being hard of hearing and being deaf (Ross, 1982). In schools for the deaf, many children are potentially hard of hearing but functionally deaf (Wedenberg and Wedenberg, 1970).

Language Deficit

Hard of hearing children with even minimal hearing loss are generally behind in school. Table 1-1 provides data on the impact of varying degrees of hearing loss upon language subtest scores of the Stanford Achievement Test. Children with less than 15 dB hearing loss, including even those with unilateral impairment, were retarded in knowing the meaning of words and paragraphs and in the selection of appropriate language forms from options presented to them. As hearing loss increased, the academic deficits increased. These findings are particularly impressive in that the community of people from which these children were drawn was at a higher-than-average socioeconomic level (Quigley and Thomure, 1968).

A recent study of the academic performance of hard of hearing students in a large Utah school district revealed similar findings. First, second, third, and fourth grade students with mild hearing losses were academically behind their normal hearing peers. Deficits existed in arithmetic problem solving, math concepts, vocabulary, and reading comprehension (Fig. 1-6). The test was the widely accepted Iowa Test

Table 1-1. Differences between Expected Performance and Actual Performance of Hard of Hearing Students on Various Subtests of the Stanford Achievement Test

Hearing threshold level (better ear)	Number	IQ	Word meaning	Paragraph meaning	Language	Subtest average
Less than 15 dB	59	105.14	−1.04	−1.04	−0.78	−0.73
15–25 dB	37	100.81	−1.40	−.86	−1.16	−1.11
27–40 dB	6	103.50	−3.40	−1.78	−1.95	−2.31
41–55 dB	9	97.89	−3.84	−2.54	−2.93	−3.08
56–70 dB	5	92.40	−2.78	−2.20	−3.52	−2.78
Total group	116	102.56	−1.66	−0.90	−1.30	−1.25

From Quigley, S., and Thomure, F. (1968). Some effects of hearing impairment on school performance. Springfield, IL: Illinois Office of Public Instruction. Reprinted by permission.

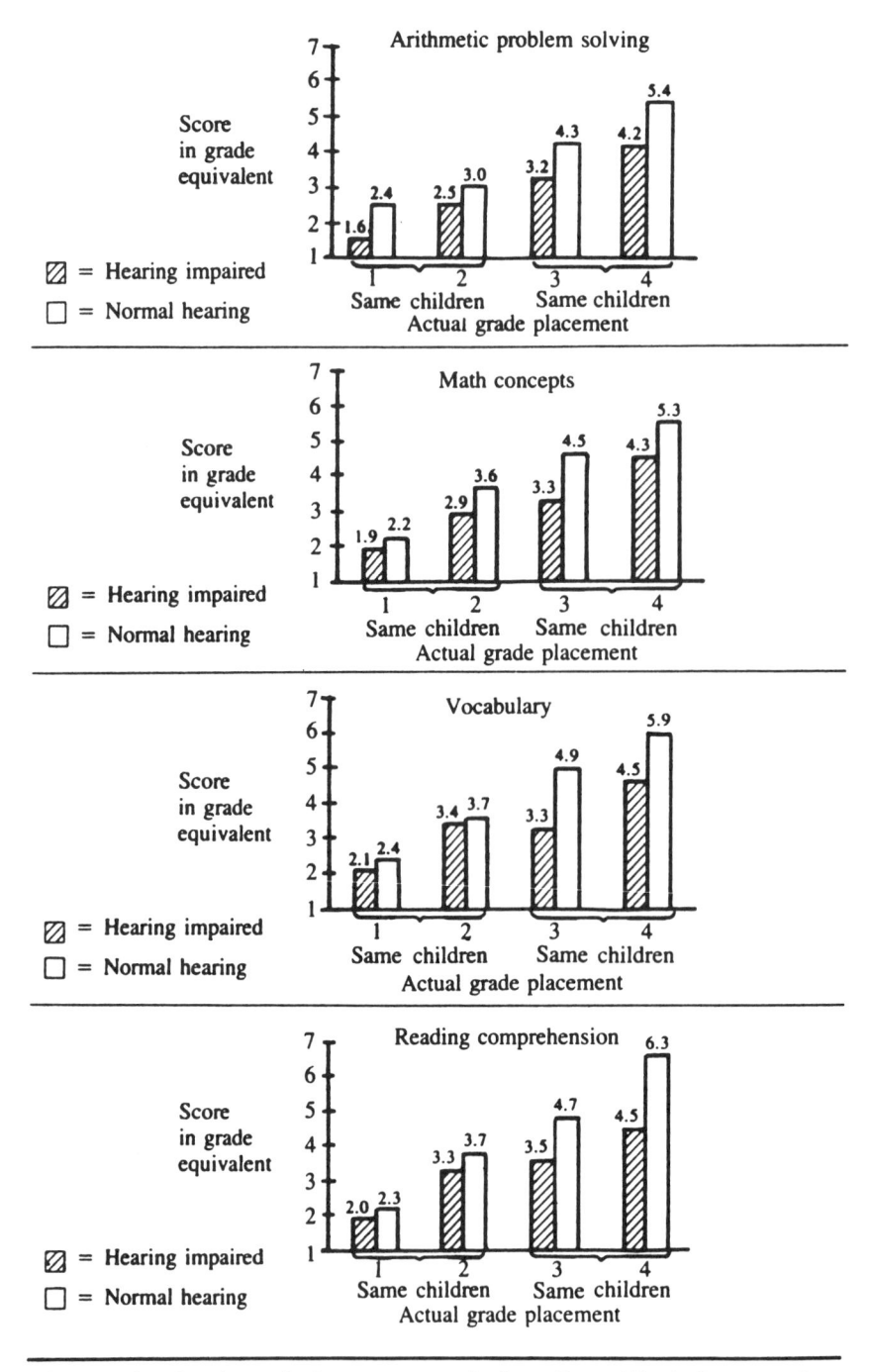

Figure 1-6. Grade equivalent scores on the Iowa Test of Basic Concepts for normal-hearing and mildly hearing-impaired youngsters. From Blair, J., et al. (1985). The effects of mild sensorineural hearing loss on academic performance of young school-age children. *The Volta Review, 87,* p. 90. Copyright 1985 by the Alexander Graham Bell Association for the Deaf, Inc. Reprinted by permission.

of Basic Concepts. The sample consisted of 48 students. Twenty-four students with hearing losses of 20 to 45 dB were the experimental group. For each student with hearing loss, a normal hearing student was chosen (24 in all) as a control. Each of the 24 pairs was matched by age, sex, socioeconomic status, and school experience. All children had normal intelligence. Note that the students with hearing losses were not behind grade level, according to national norms, but they were behind their normal hearing peers. Only four of the students with hearing impairment used hearing aids. Two of these students were not behind their normal hearing peers (Blair, Peterson, and Viehweg, 1985).

Educational Audiology Association

The Educational Audiology Association (EAA) was recently organized to "facilitate the delivery of a full spectrum of audiological services to children with auditory impairments in educational settings." The 1985 Educational Audiology Directory, the first publication of the EAA, (1) identifies approximately 1,500 audiologists interested in school children with hearing losses and (2) describes the status of educational audiology in the United States and, to a very minor extent, Canada. Membership in the EAA is open to audiologists, speech-language pathologists, educators of the hearing impaired, and persons of related fields. A quarterly EAA newsletter is published. Meetings are held in conjunction with the national conventions of the American Speech-Language-Hearing Association and the Alexander Graham Bell Association for the Deaf. Further information on the EAA can be obtained by writing Dr. James C. Blair, Department of Communicative Disorders, Utah State University, Logan, UT 84322-1000.

Chapter 2

Hearing Considerations

CASE STUDY

LB is a 5 year old kindergarten boy. Like many of his peers he has had many earaches in his young life. He also is one of tens of thousands of children who have tiny tubes in their eardrums. Medical ear specialists insert these tubes to take the place of nonfunctioning eustachian tubes in children. A functioning tube is needed so that air pressure in front of and behind an eardrum is equalized. Otherwise, the eardrum will not respond effectively to incoming sounds. The artificial tubes are removed once the eustachian tubes function again.

LB's kindergarten teacher wonders if she has other students who also have nonfunctioning eustachian tubes. It seems to her that at any one time several children in her class do not hear everything she says. Perhaps they need tubes in their ears too. She wonders what a teacher can do to identify children with ear problems.

The school district in which LB is enrolled has an audiologist, several speech-language pathologists, and several school nurses. They conduct a large-scale hearing conservation program, including screening all kindergarten children for hearing problems at the beginning of the school year. Many children with blocked eustachian tubes are identified at that time and referred through parents to their family physicians. If children develop ear problems at other times of the year, their needs are not so readily apparent. There are just too many children for the audiologist and speech-language pathologists to follow up. The school nurses also do not have time to closely monitor all kinds of health problems, unless children complain to them.

When a blocked eustachian tube is not referred for medical attention, a child often develops serous otitis media (middle ear inflammation). This is a condition in which fluid from the lining of the middle ear takes the place of the air behind the eardrum. Fluid in the ears keeps children from hearing well and often develops into a more serious hearing loss. In many instances, there is little or no pain associated with serous otitis media, and that keeps children's needs from being quickly reported.

Almost from birth, LB has had repeated bouts of otitis media. Usually his ears have filled with fluid. Once, the fluid thickened and he developed what his doctor called a "glue ear." During part of his young life he had a rather continual middle ear inflammation. At other times, his ears have been all right. The total impact of LB's fluctuating ear problems has been devastating to his learning and has put him behind in school.

LB's teacher wants to learn about ear problems and hearing loss. She has read that there is a high prevalence of hearing problems among school children, particularly those in kindergarten and the lower grades. She has a lot of questions about LB's condition and hearing loss in general. What are the chief causes of hearing loss in childhood? Where in the ear do the problems occur? At what age do they occur? What is included in a hearing conservation program? What techniques are used to identify ear problems, hearing loss, and listening problems? What is the role of a classroom teacher in all of this?

HEARING

Environmental Sound

Hearing is perhaps a person's most versatile and valuable sense. Uniquely designed, it personalizes or decodes for people much of the world in which they live. It reaches behind, under, up above, around corners, through walls, and over hills, bringing in the crackling of a distant campfire, the bubbling of a nearby stream, the closing of a door, the message of a voice, the myriad of sound that identifies surrounding events.

Sound fills people's environment. It is in a house, under a tree, on a bus, beside a stream, over a city, near a field, in place after place. It encompasses a storm, a symphony, a speech, a splash, a commotion, a call, or a kiss. Sound includes a roar, a clatter, a clang, a rustle, a squeak, and a murmur.

In keeping people in contact with their enviornment, hearing is unique in that it is multidirectional and continual. In contrast, the eyes perceive a narrower segment of the surrounding environment at any one time. The eyes also close, whereas the ears do not. Both hearing and vision, however, are the lead senses of people. Antenna-like, they intercept sounds and sights to keep a person in "touch" with the close and distant environment.

Language, Thought, and Speech

The hearing of sound also enables people to learn language during childhood. Environmental sounds and sights and people's comments about them become associated in the child's brain. With repeated exposure to experience and spoken descriptions of it, children learn to understand and express original ideas and feelings in the language of people around them. For example, one 4 year old spontaneously said, "My tummy hurts so much it's going to cry its heart out." "He's a househopper. If he was on the pavement, he'd be called a pavement-hopper. If he was on the grass, he'd be called a grasshopper like he usually is."

Hearing enables children to learn to express their thoughts and feelings in articulate speech. To learn to speak, children need hearing to compare how they say words and sentences with the way people around them say words and sentences. For example, a boy may try to say *candy,* which he hears another family member say, and hear himself say *ay, dany, tandy,* and finally *candy,* as his speech patterns become more articulate over a span of years. Having learned to articulate *candy* correctly, hearing informs the boy whether or not he is continuing to say it correctly, and does so into and throughout adulthood.

Reading, Writing, and Living

Only when the basics of language are acquired can children learn to read and write. The acquisition of reading and writing is normally a process of adapting the language basically acquired while learning to listen and speak. The beginning years of school are designed in large part to aid children in making this transfer so they can communicate meanings by use of alphabet letters as well as speech sounds.

Hearing also contributes to the manner in which children plan their lives, cope with problems, and organize experience. It has a pervasive influence that affects personal adjustment, social competence, and vocational fulfillment. Hearing causes children to perceive the world, conceptualize experience, describe events, and anticipate the future in a different light than if hearing were absent or not utilized.

HEARING MECHANISM

Hearing is possible because within each side of the head is a masterpiece of creation called an ear. The human ear, or hearing mechanism, is delicately arranged so that almost infinitesimally small amounts of sound can be received and recorded in the brain. It also has a built-in system to protect itself somewhat from unusually loud and unwanted sound.

Parts of the Ear

The hearing mechanism can be divided into four parts (see Fig. 2–1):

1. The outer ear, with its protruding flap (auricle) for collecting sound and its ear canal (auditory meatus) through which sound passes to reach other parts of the hearing mechanism.

2. The middle ear, or air space, which contains a system of levers (malleus, incus, stapes), called ossicles, which conduct the sound from the eardrum (tympanic membrane) to the oval window leading to the inner ear.

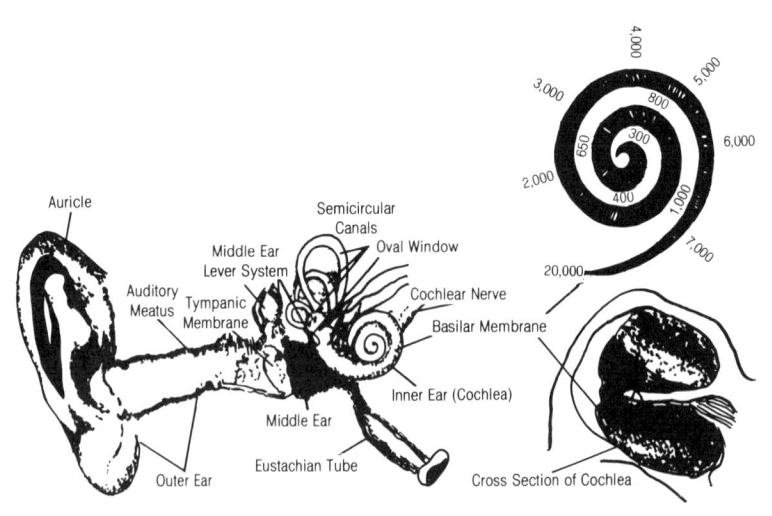

Figure 2–1. Parts of the ear. From Berg, F. (1971). *Breakthrough for the hard of hearing child* (p. 3). Smithfield, UT: Ear Publication. Reprinted by permission.

3. The inner ear, or fluid space, which contains organs for hearing (cochlea) and balance (semicircular canals), and which changes vibrational energy of incoming sound into electrical (nerve) impulses.

4. The cochlear nerve, with its many thousands of electrical cells (with fibers) running side by side from the organ of hearing to numerous relay stations before reaching the auditory centers of the brain.

The outer and middle parts of the ears are often called the conductive mechanism; the inner and nerve portions, the perceptive (sensorineural) mechanism.

Simplified Description of How We Hear

A simplified description of how sound gets to the brain, as shown in Figure 2-2.

1. Sound waves striking the eardrum operate the three smallest bones of the body (the ossicles, known as the hammer, the anvil, and the stirrup).

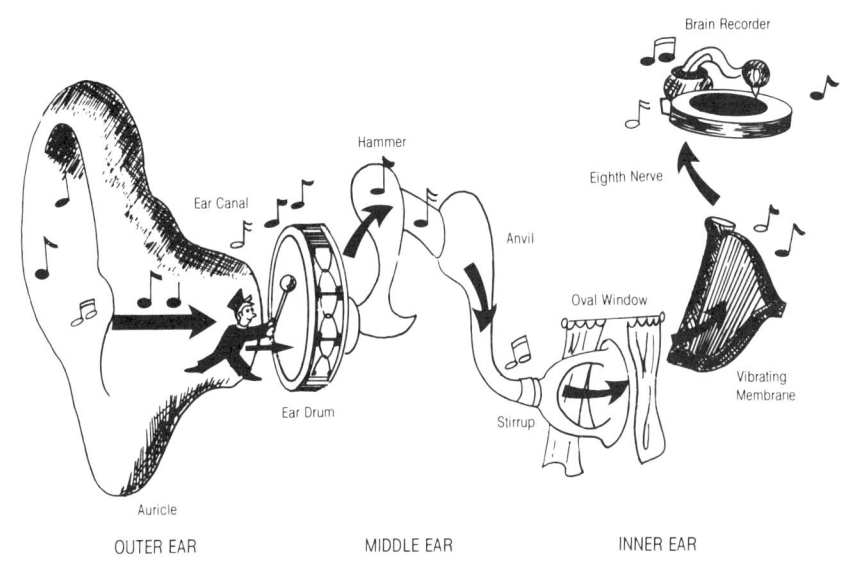

Figure 2-2. How we hear. From Sonotone color poster. Ossining, NY: Sonotone International. Adapted by permission.

2. The stirrup, in turn, vibrates the oval window—a thin membrane stretched across the entrance to the inner ear.
3. Movement of the oval window is passed on to the cochlea, the organ of hearing, which "feels" the mechanical movements caused by sound waves.
4. This vibrating membrane, containing 25,000 tiny hair cells, analyzes the vibrations received and sends the results to the brain via the eighth, or hearing, nerve.

DESCRIPTION OF HEARING LOSS

Description of Hearing Loss

Children can hear effectively when all structures of the hearing mechanism are fully operational. A hearing loss occurs when a pathologic condition exists in an ear owing to a disease or other cause. Each specific cause of hearing loss damages one or more parts of the ear before birth, with birth, or after birth. Hearing loss is classified as conductive, sensorineural, or mixed, depending on the location of the pathologic condition (Fig. 2–3). The resulting hearing loss may be slight to total and may occur in one ear or both ears. The degree of loss may stay the same, progress, or fluctuate. Sometimes hearing loss is but one of several handicaps resulting from a particular causative agent.

Causes of Hearing Loss

The most common cause of hearing loss among elementary school children is otitis media (middle ear inflammation). The majority of all children have had at least one episode of otitis media by the age of 6 years. Serous otitis media (fluid within the middle ear) occurs often when the eustachian tube is blocked (Fig. 2–4). It is especially common among children in kindergarten through the fourth grade and is resistant to medical treatment. Otitis media can also be chronic or recurrent. Temporary or permanent conductive hearing loss in one or both ears results from otitis media.

As children get older, and especially by the time they are teenagers, there is particular concern with their acquiring sensorineural hearing loss due to exposure to intense sounds. A noise-induced hearing loss can occur instantaneously from a sudden extremely intense sound, or gradually from prolonged intense sound. Many secondary school students have hearing loss in both ears caused by exposure to firecrackers, gunfire, motorcycles, farm tractors, power mowers, snowmobiles, rock music, and other causes of intense sound (Fig. 2–5).

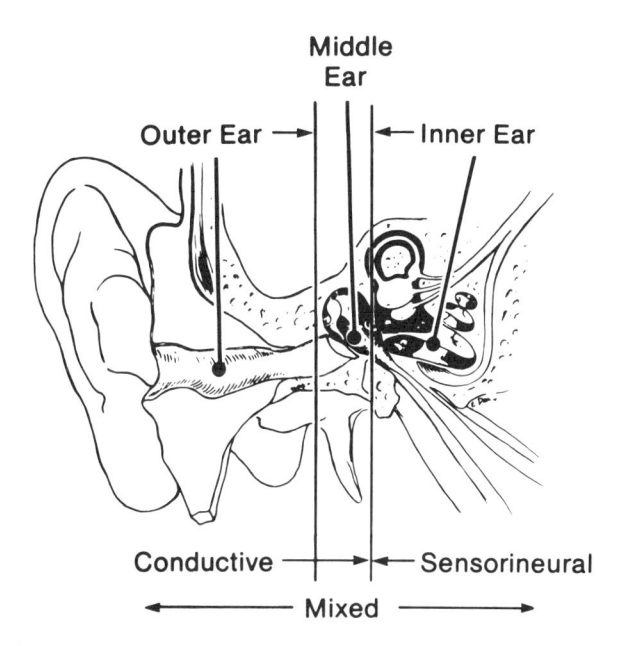

Figure 2-3. Three types of hearing loss. From Roeser, R., and Price, D. (1972). Audiometric and impedance measures. In R. Roeser and M. Downs (Eds.), *Auditory disorders in school children* (2nd ed., p. 81). New York: Thieme-Stratton. Copyright 1981 by Thieme-Stratton, Inc. Reprinted by permission.

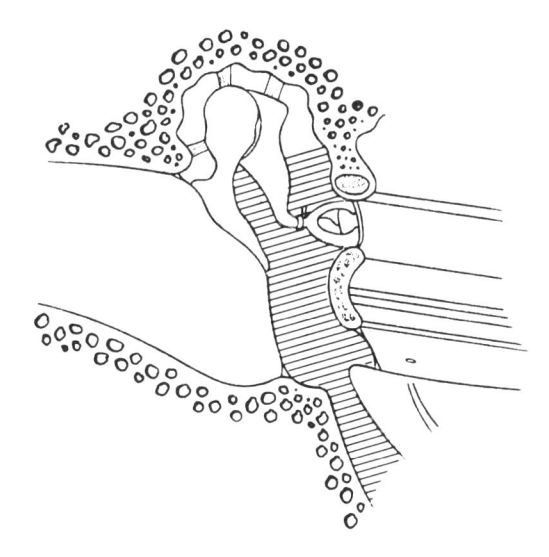

Figure 2-4. Fluid in serous (secretory) otitis media. From Goodhill, V., and Brockman, S. (1979). Secretory otitis media. In V. Goodhill (Ed.), *Diseases, deafness and dizziness* (p. 310). Hagerstown, MD: Harper & Row. Copyright 1979 by Harper & Row, Inc. Reprinted by permission.

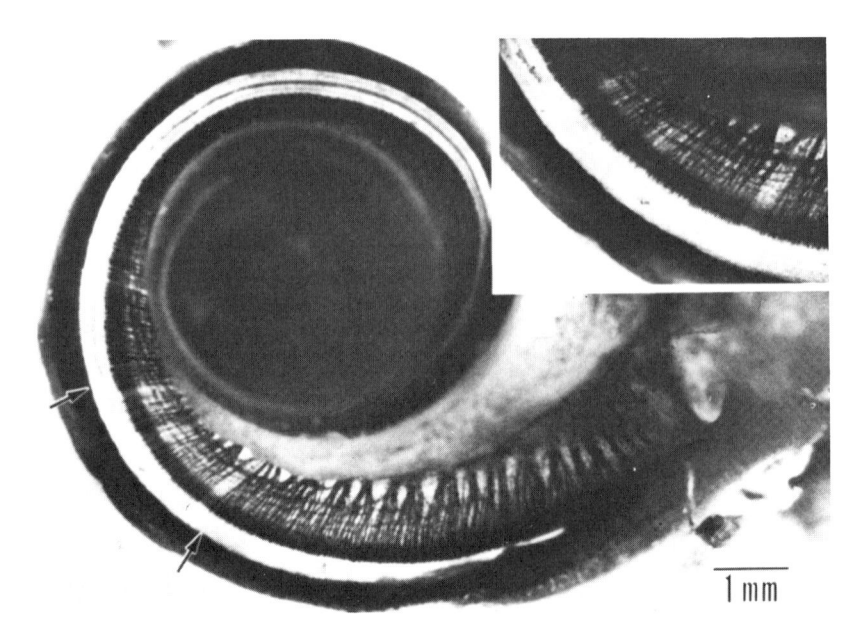

Figure 2-5. Damage (between arrows) in left cochlea due to noise exposure. From Johnsson, L., and Hawkins, J. (1976). Degeneration patterns in human ears exposed to noise. *Transactions of the American Otolaryngological Society, 64,* 52–66. Reprinted by permission.

In special education classes many children have mongolism, called Down's syndrome. These children have been born learning disabled from genetically caused brain damage. Mongoloid children also have malformation or destruction of ossicles in their middle ears, causing hearing loss in both ears.

A list of conditions and causes of temporary or permanent hearing loss among children appears below. Often something that causes hearing loss also causes another problem that is not listed.

1. Auricle malformed from birth
2. Ear canal closed by inflammation, fluid or scar
3. Eardrum ruptured by object inserted in ear canal
4. Middle ear filled with fluid because of blocked eustachian tube
5. Middle ear and inner ear damaged by chronic middle ear infection
6. Middle ear obstructed by cholesteatoma (growth) from skin that passes through eardrum (Fig. 2–6)
7. One or more parts of ear not developed because of genetic defect

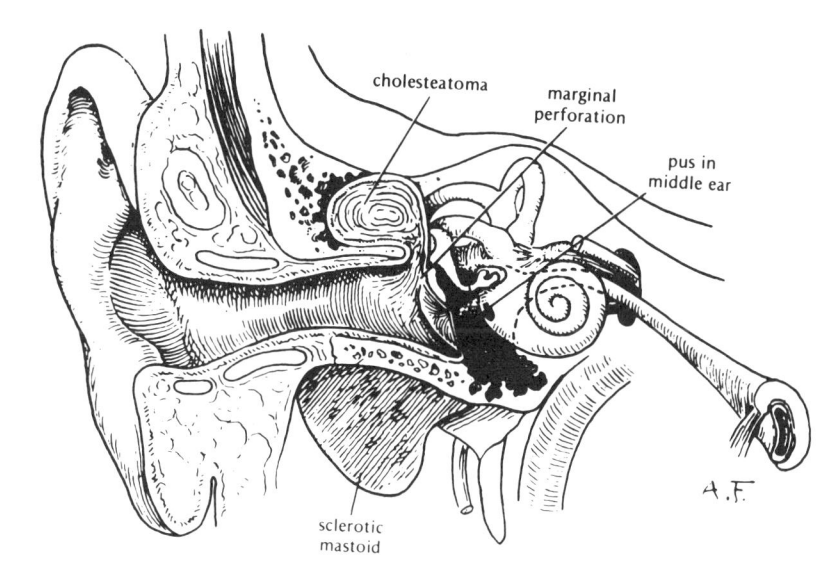

Figure 2-6. A cholesteatoma next to the eardrum. From Davis, H. (1979). Abnormal hearing and deafness. In H. Davis and S. R. Silverman (Eds.), *Hearing and deafness* (p. 111). New York: Holt, Rinehart, & Winston. Copyright 1947, 1960, 1970 by Holt, Rinehart, & Winston, Inc. Reprinted by permission of CBS College Publishing.

8. Middle ear ossicles disconnected or cochlear structures destroyed by blows to the head
9. Cochlear cells lost because of prolonged life-saving toxic medication
10. Cochlear damaged by very intense noise or prolonged exposure to loud sound
11. Cochlear damaged by mumps, meningitis, viral influenza, rubella, syphilis, or blood incompatibility between mother and fetus
12. Auditory nerve progressively damaged by developing tumor

HEARING CONSERVATION

Medical Care

Like other structures of the body, the ear is amenable to medical or surgical help. The family physician or pediatrician, for example, may stop an earache and eliminate infection of the middle ear. The otologist (medical ear specialist) may repair an eardrum that has burst and even rebuild a middle ear wasted away by prolonged infection (Fig. 2–7). The preventive contribution of the public health nurse in inoculating

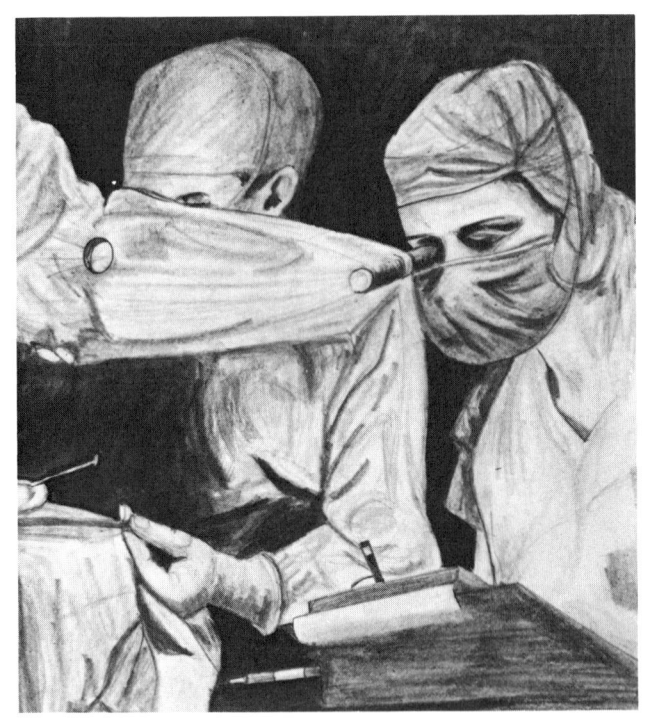

Figure 2-7. Microsurgery of the ear. From Papanella, M. (1971). *Columbus Dispatch Sunday Magazine.* Adapted by permission.

against disease and teaching ear hygiene should be recognized also. In the process of these medical or health endeavors, certain cases of hearing impairment may be prevented, others reversed, and still others at least lessened in degree. Consideration of cause, pathologic condition, treatment, and hearing improvement is illustrated through several examples in Table 2–1.

As in other medical branches, otological care has improved dramatically in recent years, and even more impressive advances may lie ahead. New medicines may control or eliminate infection more permanently. Other ear and middle ear surgery may improve. Tumors may be identified sooner so that the success rate of brain surgery is increased. There may be a breakthrough in the repair of pathologic conditions of the cochlea. Currently, cochlear operations are not performed because the inner ear is difficult to reach, exceedingly intricate, and very sensitive to surgical damage.

Table 2-1. Possible Hearing Conservation Considerations

Cause	Pathologic condition	Treatment	Hearing improvement in decibels (dB)
Wax secreted or object inserted into ear canal	Ear canal becomes plugged, impeding passage of sound to ear drum	Physician removes wax or obstruction	20 dB loss originally, normal hearing after wax removal
Allergy causes swelling, which closes eustachian tube	Air leaves middle ear and fluid enters, impeding passage of sound through middle ear	Physician prescribes decongestant drug, which relieves swelling, opens tube and ventilates ear	30 dB originally; normal hearing after adminstration of decongestant drug
Previous condition untreated	Fluid thickens, later choleosteatoma forms, impeding passage of sound through middle ear and threatening life	Otologist removes cholesteatoma and rebuilds middle ear	60 dB loss originally; 20 dB after operation
Mother contracts rubella (German measles) during early pregnancy	Child born with much of cochlea gone, interfering with transfer of sound to nerve impulses	Otologist cannot help; birth could have been aborted	Permanent 75 dB loss
Characteristic of hearing loss transmitted genetically to child	Child born with even less cochlea	Otologist cannot help; genetic counseling beforehand might have prevented conception of child	Permanent 85 dB loss

Audiological Assistance

During the Second World War the audiology specialty was initiated in the United States. Audiology is the nonmedical discipline, body of knowledge, and techiques and activities for caring for the hearing impaired. By 1985 there were 6700 certified audiologists in the country. Many audiologists assist otologists in diagnosing pathologic conditions of the ear and in evaluating the effects of medical and surgical treatment. About 400 audiologists work in the schools and are called educational audiologists. They have comprehensive hearing conservation responsibilities, beginning with identifying children with hearing loss and pathologic conditions of the ear. Most school districts do not employ audiologists but do employ speech-language pathologists, who screen children for hearing loss. State health and crippled children's agencies also provide hearing identification assistance to school districts as needed.

When a school child is suspected of having a pathologic condition of the ear, the parents or guardians are informed. If a school district does not employ an audiologist or does not receive services from an audiologist, the parents or primary caregivers then have the responsibility to arrange for audiological evaluation at a hearing center (Fig. 2–8). School district services for children with hearing loss are enhanced by the employment of educational audiologists because they understand the characteristics and needs of these children and can provide immediate testing and technical assistance with classroom acoustics, hearing aids, and FM equipment.

Hearing screening and medical referral programs have been operative in the public schools for 50 years. Recent federal regulations stipulate that all children with possible handicap receive free diagnostic evaluation through state crippled children's programs. Also, Public Law 94–142 states that a child whose educational performance is adversely affected by a hearing loss must be identified, evaluated, and assured a free and appropriate education.

School nurses also provide support for hearing identification programs. There are nearly 40,000 school nurses in the 16,000 school districts of this country. In addition to the "band-aid" type of work, they serve as counselors, detectors of abnormal problems, and health educa-

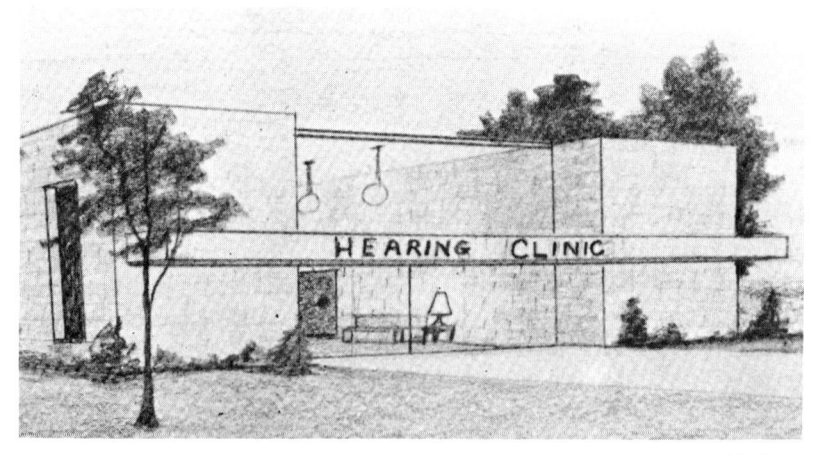

Figure 2-8. Hearing center for evaluating and assisting persons with hearing loss. From Berg, F. (1971). *Breakthrough for the hard of hearing child* (p. 24). Smithfield, UT: Ear Publication. Reprinted by permission.

tors. The school nurse is a pivotal professional between the student, teacher, parent, and other health personnel in translating and integrating medical findings and recommendations.

Identification Instruments

Hearing screening programs in the schools involve the use of an otoscope, an impedance tympanometer, and an audiometer. A fourth hearing screening instrument, the acoustic otoscope, has recently been developed. The otoscope, impedance tympanometer, and acoustic otoscope will be described in this chapter. The audiometer will be explained in the third chapter. The role of the classroom teacher with these instruments will be discussed.

Otoscope

An otoscope is an instrument that provides lighted magnification for examining the ear, particularly the eardrum. With an otoscope, the audiologist should look for blockage of the ear canal, obvious inflammatory processes, and ear discharge. The identification of any of these ear problems by the audiologist should lead to immediate medical referral. On the basis of lack of training in otoscopy, however, the audiologist will miss many ear problems that would be apparent to an otologist or other physician.

The otoscope used by a medical doctor is called a pneumatic otoscope (Fig. 2–9). It includes provision for creating a positive or negative air pressure in the ear canal to test the mobility of the eardrum. Acute otitis media can be recognized by the audiologist using a simple otoscope because the eardrum will be red and bulging. The otologist with a pneumatic otoscope, however, will also be able to determine the mobility of the eardrum, which with acute otitis media will be abnormally minimal. The immobility of the eardrum may be the more important of the two clues to acute otitis media. Within the middle ear, acute otitis is characterized by severe infection and the presence of bacteria. There is pus in the middle ear, and earache, and there will be drainage into the ear canal if the eardrum bursts. It is important that this problem be identified and treated in its early stages.

The pneumatic otoscope is also used by the otologist for detecting serous otitis media, which is persistence of fluid in the middle ear. This condition often causes educational delay, because both ears are involved, and the symptoms of the abnormality often do not exist. By the time the fluid is recognized, it is usually thick and tenacious. Called "glue ear" by physicians, the middle ear is full of this material, and hearing is definitely impaired. Lack of mobility of the eardrum will be detected with the pneumatic otoscope.

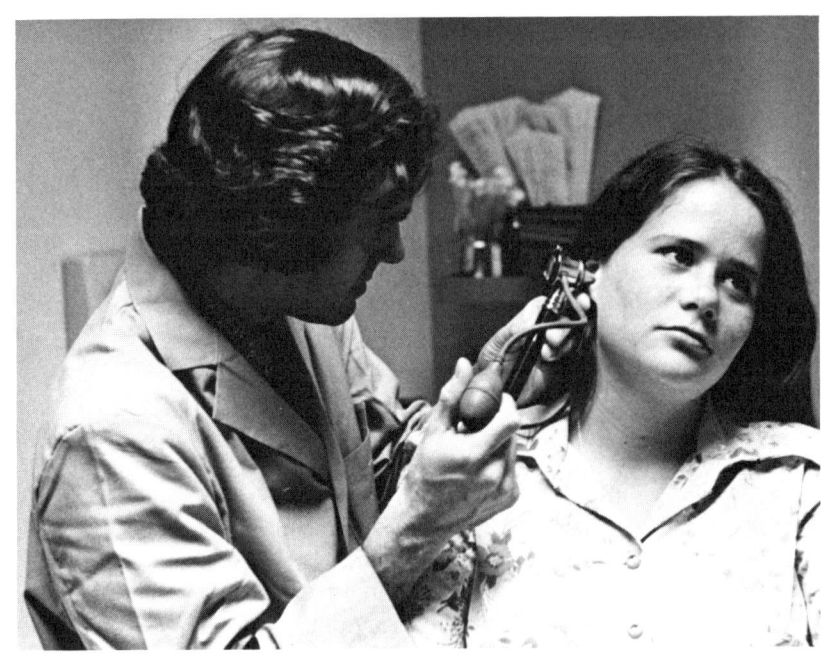

Figure 2-9. Pneumatic otoscope in use. From Goodhill, V. (1979). Ear examination. In V. Goodhill (Ed.), *Diseases, deafness, and dizziness.* (p. 92) Hagerstown, MD: Harper & Row. Copyright 1979 by Harper & Row, Inc. Reprinted by permission.

The classroom teacher can also learn to use a simple otoscope to see obvious ear abnormalities but must be cautioned against the practice. First, there is the problem of keeping the otoscope sterilized. Second, the teacher will be busy with other responsibilities. Third, the teacher can request the assistance of the audiologists or speech-language pathologists for simple otoscopic checks. Fourth, the teacher will not have sufficient depth of training not to be liable to possible lawsuits.

Teachers, however, need to be aware of the value of the otoscope in a school screening program. They should also be on the alert for symptoms of outer and middle ear problems. Children with pathologic conditions of the ear may have upper respiratory infection, fever, an itching or aching ear, or not feel well. Teachers may note ear drainage and a foul odor associated with acute (brief severe) and chronic (long-standing) otitis media. They should realize that surgical drainage of the middle ear and the insertion of tubes in the eardrum are controversial medical procedures, but that these procedures appear to improve the function of the middle ear and decrease the number of infections. They should be aware that prescribed antihistamines and anticongestants are often but not always helpful. Teachers need to be sensitive to the strain that recurrent otitis media, both acute and serous, can place on families and the health care system. Teachers can appreciate the value of the otoscope in identifying problems of the middle ear by looking at colored slides of normal and pathological eardrums that are of particular value to physicians.

The actual diagnosis of pathologic conditions is the province of the physician, particularly the otologist. Under no circumstances should anyone other than the physician attempt to remove ear wax or a foreign body from the ear canal or insert a hairpin or cotton-tipped applicator or the like into it. Also, extreme care should be taken to not push material further into the ear canal during visual inspection. Otherwise, the ear canal may become occluded, or the eardrum perforated, or the material pushed into and damage the middle ear. Otologists have found beans, cotton, crumpled tissue, matchsticks, toothpicks, and other foreign objects in the ear canal. These objects and impacted earwax, upon removal, may reveal further ear abnormalities. Notwithstanding the skill and tools of even the otologist, safe removal of foreign bodies impacted deep in the ear canal is impossible without anesthesia, particularly in a child.

Impedance Meter

The impedance meter is the second instrument used for identifying ear or hearing problems. Both the audiologist and the speech pathologist use this instrument in the schools, and physicians use it in medical facilities. Of particular interest to teachers are tympanograms (graphs) of the mobility or compliance of the tympanic membranes (eardrums). Together with other measures obtained with this instrument and other instruments like the pneumatic otoscope, tympanograms enable specialists to know what, if anything, might be wrong with the middle ear and associated structures, without surgically operating to inspect the middle ear. Progress in medical and surgical treatment of the ears can also be monitored by obtaining repeated tympanograms.

Both diagnostic and screening impedance meters are available. Screening meters are used more often in the schools because of their lower cost and their capability of obtaining basic information very rapidly (Fig. 2–10). Some audiologists prefer using only diagnostic impedance meters, emphasizing their high reliability. Using impedance equipment does not require a special test environment. Also, test results are obtained directly and do not depend upon voluntary responses of

32 Facilitating Classroom Listening

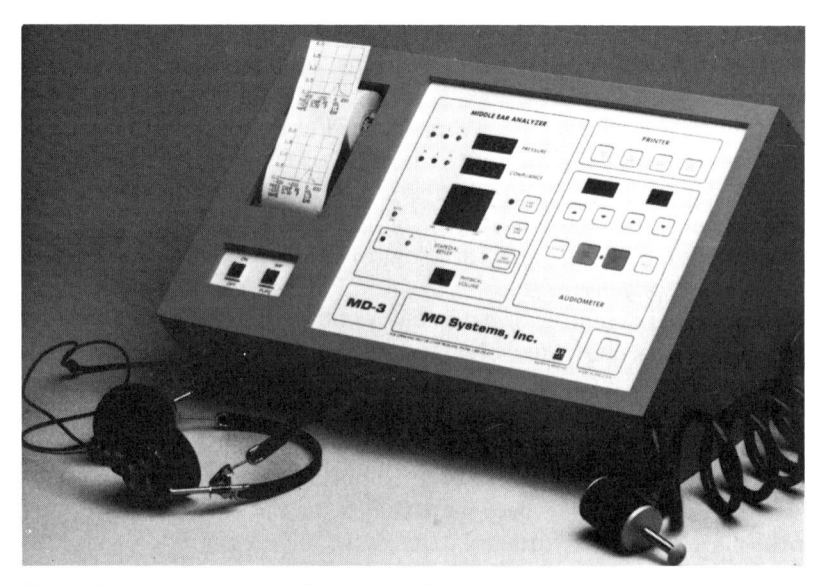

Figure 2-10. A screening instrument for obtaining tympanograms and supportive information on ear pathology and hearing loss. From G. A. Levow advertisement on MD screening system. West Newton MA. Reprinted by permission.

children. Probe tips of various sizes are used to provide a necessary air seal in the ear canal. Sound reflected from the eardrum is measured and graphed while air pressure is varied.

Each tympanogram is an interaction of the mobility (0 to 10 scale) of the eardrum and varying air pressure (-300 to $+200$ mm of H_2O) around atmospheric pressure (0). Figure 2-11 shows a tympanogram for a normal ear and the four common types (As, Ad, B, and C) of abnormal tympanograms. Table 2-2 describes possible problems that give rise to these typical tympanograms. The specific tympanogram, combined with other measures, helps the otologist predict the specific problem prior to medical or surgical treatment.

An impedance meter is often as good a tool as the pneumatic otoscope in determining the status of the middle ear. It is now widely used by otologists as a complementary diagnostic tool to the pneumatic otoscope. Diagnostic information obtained by using the one tool confirms data from using the other tool. The impedance meter is also a device that the educational audiologist and the speech-language pathologist can use effectively.

Knowing what a normal tympanogram looks like and what abnormal tympanograms look like provides teachers with ownership of information on the status of the conductive hearing mechanisms of students

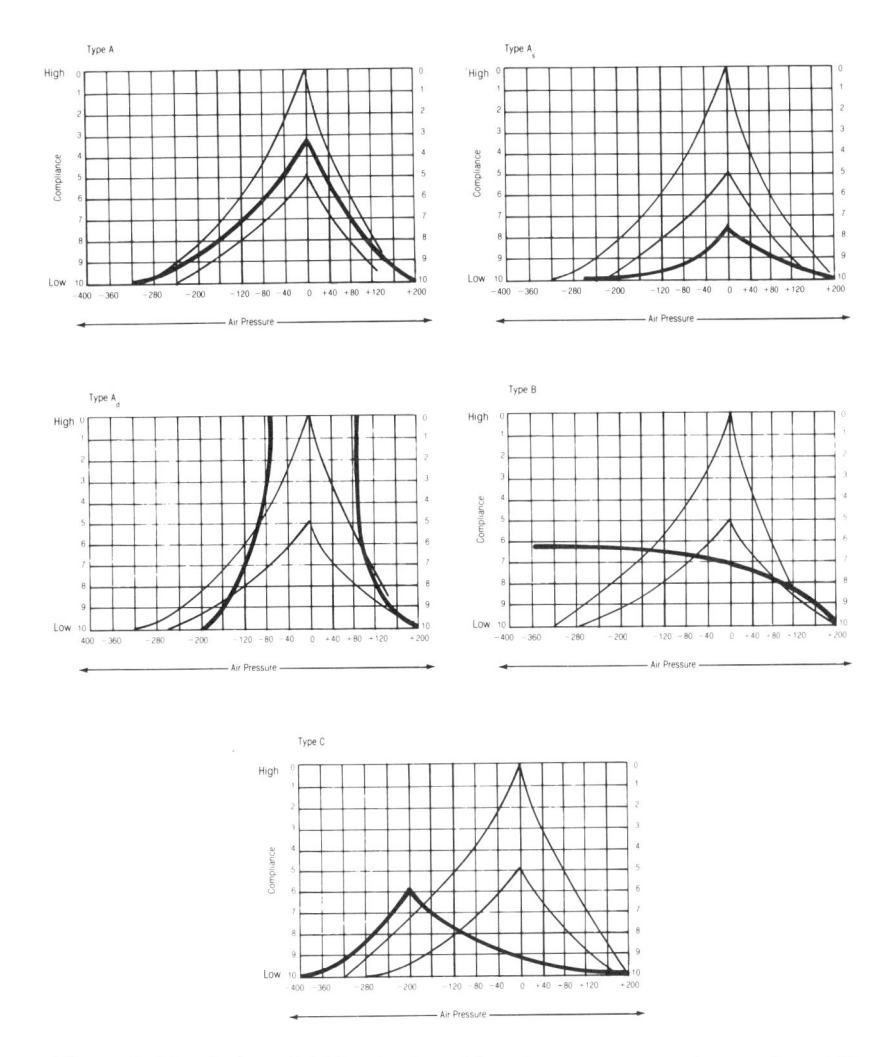

Figure 2–11. Left to right beginning at top: tympanogram of normal ear (A) and tympanograms of pathological ears (As, Ad, B, and C). From Jerger, J. (1970). Clinical experience with impedance audiometry. *Archives of Otolaryngology, 92,* 311–324. Reprinted by permission.

Table 2-2. Possible Ear Problems Contributing to Typical Tympanograms

Type	Mobility/pressure	Possible problems
A	Normal at 0	None
As	Limited (stiff) at 0	Heavily scarred or ossified eardrum
Ad	Too much at 0	Flaccid eardrum or middle ear bones disconnected
B	Limited at any value	Ear canal totally occluded, hole in eardrum (could be ventilating tube), fluid in middle ear or eardrum is severely retracted, adhesive tissue may restrict movement of middle ear bones, or congenital middle ear malformation may exist
C	Near normal at −200 or below	Eustachian tube does not function, fluid may be in the middle ear

in their classes. Teachers may then become more active in facilitating the identification of ear problems and hearing loss and medical referral as necessary. Being able to interpret common tympanograms also gives teachers a base upon which to make further study of pathologic conditions and their impact upon teaching and learning.

Acoustic Otoscope

The recently developed acoustic otoscope provides the schools with a simple, relatively inexpensive option to screening for serous otitis media. With a touch of a button, this hand-held instrument delivers a loud sound into the ear canal, which reflects from the eardrum and is measured by a microphone (Fig. 2–12). Unlike the impedance meter, no air pressure seal is involved.

This device is applicable for all persons over 6 months of age. Crying does not affect results. Middle ear fluid can be detected in seven of eight persons who have it. Two of three persons who do not have fluid can also be identified.

The response relies on the principle of partial cancellation of the incident sound by sound reflected from the eardrum. The probe sound can be described as a chirping bird. Replaceable plastic tips and a replaceable battery are used. A simple calibration test assures accurate readings.

The device gives visible readings on two scales, reflectivity and length (Fig. 2–13). *Reflectivity* is a number (0–9) on the vertical scale. It indicates the level of transmitted sound that is reflected from the ear drum. A reading of 9 indicates a complete reflection, and 0, minimal reflection. Research and experience show that readings of 0 to 4 usually mean that no middle ear fluid exists, and readings of 6 to 9 nearly always mean that it does exist. *Length* is a number (0 to 9) on the

Hearing Considerations 35

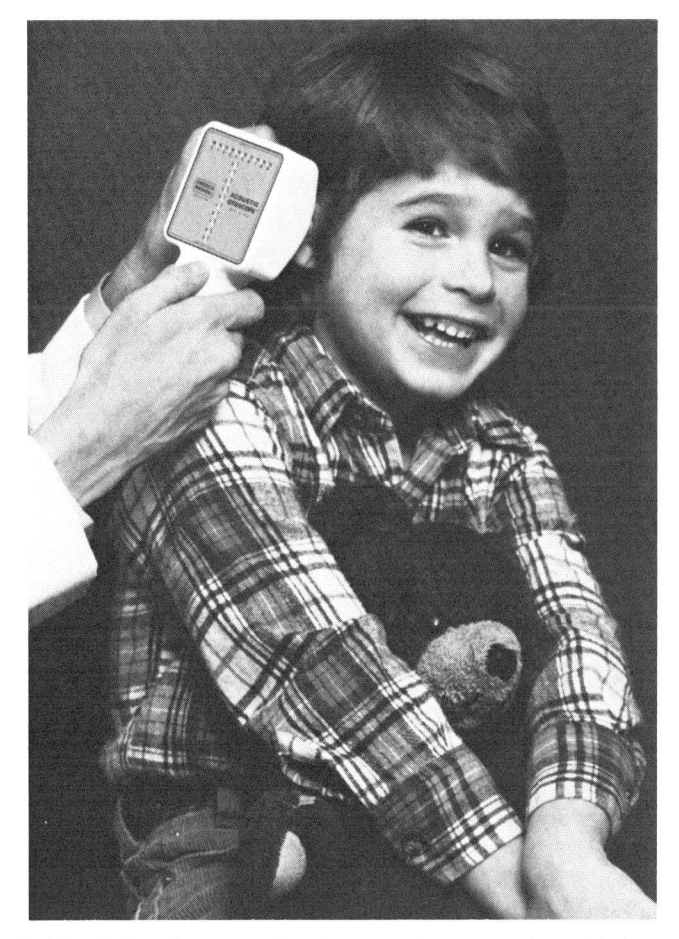

Figure 2-12. Using the acoustic otoscope to screen for middle ear fluid. From Endeco Medical, Inc. advertisement. Marion MA. Reprinted by permission.

horizontal scale. It indicates the distance between the probe tip and where the sound reflects from, usually the eardrum. A low reading often means blockage of ear wax. A high reading frequently means a sizeable eardrum perforation by which the sound is reflected from the back of the middle ear rather than from the eardrum. When the reflectivity (vertical) reading is low, the length reading should be ignored because the reflection is too weak to indicate eardrum position.

The sound produced by this device lasts only 1/10 second. A pushbutton causes it to be produced. Each time the button is pushed, the instrument will read again. On repeated testing the last reading should be

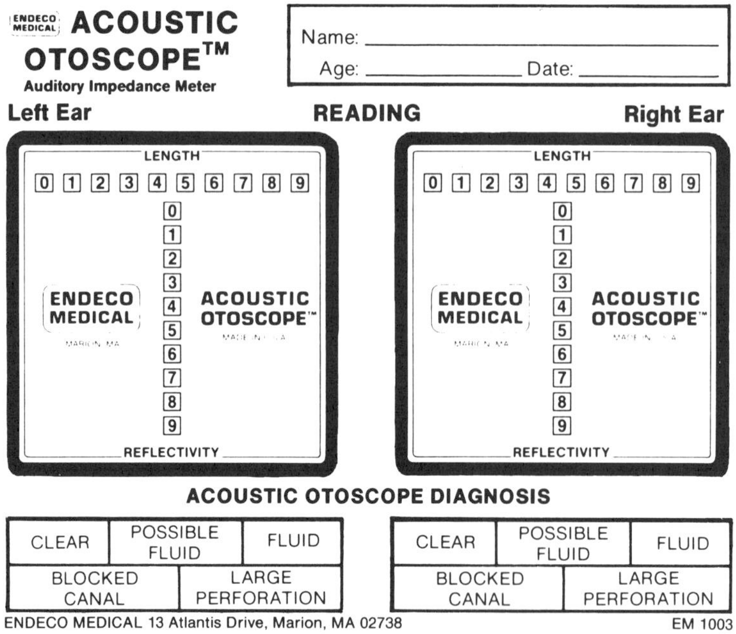

Figure 2-13. Reflectivity and length scales of the acoustic otoscope. From Endeco Medical, Inc. advertisement. Marion, MA. Reprinted by permission.

considered the most accurate. To get reproducible results, the tip (speculum) should be inserted in the ear canal and directed toward the eardrum. The instrument should be maneuvered until the highest possible reflectivity reading is achieved. The ear canal can be very narrow or nearly (90 percent) blocked and a reading still occur. Light emitting diodes are used to indicate the scale readings.

A recorder is now available for providing reflectivity versus length printouts. Any invalid test will be indicated (e.g., block or no reflection) in special print. When a series of tests are taken in a particular ear, the recorder can automatically select the highest reflectivity reading. The recorder can be set to analyze test results versus adult, child, or infant standards, and to print the diagnosis. Sample recorder outputs are shown in Figure 2-14.

The acoustic otoscope provides a school district with the capability of easily identifying children with serous otitis media. It is a device that would allow a speech-language pathologist or school nurse to rapidly and repeatedly screen school children. Classroom teachers would do well to support the purchase of the device to meet the needs of their students.

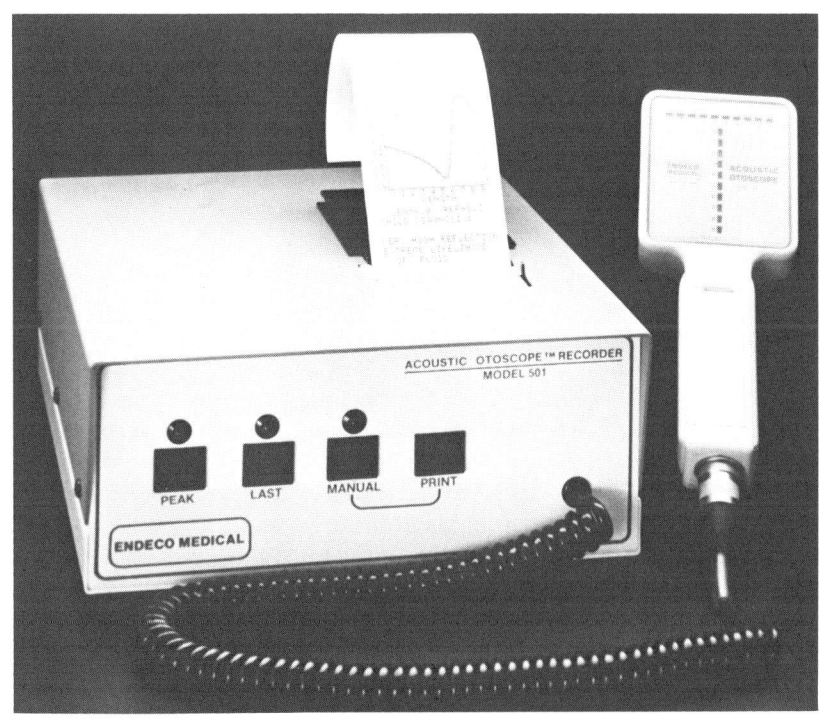

Figure 2-14. Acoustic otoscope, recorder, and printout indicating extreme likelihood of middle ear fluid. From Endeco Medical, Inc. advertisement. Marion, MA. Reprinted by permission.

SYMPTOMS OF HEARING LOSS

The hearing screening program of a school district may fail to identify a child with a hearing loss. One reason for this is that not all children are screened each year. A second reason is that a child may have a hearing loss when tested but develop a hearing problem later. A third reason is that the hearing screening program may not use equipment for detecting less than major degrees of hearing difficulty or may not have a quiet enough test environment.

The identification of ear pathologies among school children is enhanced when teachers are alerted to physical symptoms and behaviors associated with hearing loss. Physical symptoms include mouth breathing, draining ears, earaches, dizziness, and reports of ringing, buzzing, or roaring in ears. Behaviors include requests to have statements repeated, turning one side of the head toward the talker, talking too softly or loudly, showing strain while listening, concentrating attention on the lips of the talker, inattentiveness during discussions, making mistakes in taking or following directions, isolating self, being passive or tense, tiring easily, speaking incorrectly, not meeting expectations, and academic failure. When any of these symptoms or behaviors are observed in a child, the teacher should refer the child to a school audiologist or speech-language pathologist for testing, or suggest to parents that impedance and audiometric testing be considered.

SUMMARY

Hearing underlies and greatly facilitates human communication and education. However, the hearing mechanism, or ear, is susceptible to damage from many different causes. The main cause of hearing loss prior to and during the early years of school is otitis media. During the teenage years there is concern with ear damage due to exposure to intense sounds. It is essential that hearing conservation be taught and practiced in the schools, including the identification and evaluation of pathologic conditions of the ear. Children with suspected ear problems should be referred to audiologists and to physicians, including otologists.

Instruments for identification and evaluation of outer and middle ear problems used by medical and nonmedical specialists have been described in this chapter. The role of the classroom teacher in school hearing conservation programs has been explained.

FURTHER READINGS

Victor Goodhill's *Diseases, Deafness, and Dizziness* (Harper and Row, Hagerstown, MD, 1979) is a fascinating sourcebook on the medicine and surgery of the ear, with many illustrations, including colored photographs of the tympanic membrane. The book *Auditory Disorders in School Children* (Thieme-Stratton, New York, 1981), edited by Ross Roeser and Marion Downs, is a major reference on hearing conservation, particularly the chapter by Lavonne Bergstrom on medical problems and their management. Two valuable references on the anatomy, physiology, and the pathology of the ear are *Hearing and Deafness* (Holt, Rinehart, and Winston, New York, 1978), edited by Hallowell Davis and S. Richard Silverman, and *Medical Audiology* (Prentice-Hall, Englewood Cliffs, NJ, 1981), edited by Frederick Martin. The recent book *Educational Audiology for the Hard of Hearing Child* (Grune & Stratton, Orlando, FL, 1986), particularly Chapter 1 by Frederick Berg and Chapter 4 by Steven Viehweg, extend the educational and audiological information introduced in this chapter.

Chapter 3

Speech Considerations

CASE STUDY

CJ is a 10 year old hard of hearing boy who wears a hearing aid. He has had chronic middle ear disease since early childhood, notwithstanding having received otological care. He started school a year late and is not performing well in the fourth grade. His vocabulary and language constructions are like those of a first grade child. He misunderstands people, particularly when they talk fast or do not face him, or when the room is noisy. A psychologist tested CJ and reported that he is an intelligent child.

CJ has a speech problem. His speech is delayed, and many consonants sounds are omitted, substituted, or distorted. He also mispronounces many words when he tries to read.

The school district enrolls 1500 students and has a speech-language pathologist but no educational audiologist or educator of the hearing impaired. The speech-language pathologist spends part of her time in screening hearing and referring screening failures for audiological and medical assistance. The speech-language pathologist has been trained to work with the speech and language problems of persons who have normal hearing. She has had some training and experience in working with children with hearing losses.

The speech-language pathologist is assisting CJ with his speech and using remedial materials that she uses with children without hearing loss. CJ is making some improvement, but not as much as would be desirable. His parents do not have funds to hire a private speech-language pathologist. They have requested more help from the school.

CJ's fourth grade teacher has become very concerned. She would like to help with his speech but recognizes she has not been trained to do so. She wonders if she could not work with the speech-language pathologist. Perhaps together they could speed up CJ's speech and language development and improve his ability to pronounce words.

CJ's hearing aid is new. His first aid had been used by an older relative. CJ seems much more satisfied with the new aid. An audiologist in private practice selected if for him. The audiologist is checking the functioning of the aid every 3 months.

Since receiving the aid, CJ seems to hear and attend better. Neither the hearing aid nor lipreading, however, are compensating for his basic communication deficits. More specialized speech, listening, and language training are needed.

The fourth grade teacher is beginning to make a study of the sounds of speech. She has found out that while there are 26 letters of the alphabet, there are as many as 40 sounds of speech. She has found there is a special alphabet for symbolizing all the sounds of speech. It is called the International Phonetic Alphabet.

The teacher realizes she is not going to learn enough to take the place of the speech-language pathologist. She would like, however, to learn just enough to be of help. The teacher believes she could learn to recognize when the sounds of speech are misarticulated. She also believes she could take the time to reinforce correct speech behavior. She might even have time to listen as CJ practices saying difficult sounds in words in sentences. CJ's teacher could also help him pronounce words. In addition, she could spend more time in explaining what the words mean.

CJ's mother and father are anxious to help also; they just need direction. They are pleased that his teacher is trying to learn to help with speech. The speech-language pathologist has recently been given approval by her supervisor to spend more time with CJ and less time with a few other children who have less severe speech problems. She is looking for appropriate speech and listening materials and procedures to use with CJ.

BASICS OF SPEECH

Speech Mechanism

Speech is possible because of the marvelous speech mechanism of human beings. The control centers of speech are in the brain. The speech act is powered by air in the lungs. The larynx (voice box) in the neck transforms the steady flow of air from the lungs into a series of puffs, which provide the source for the voiced sounds. Constrictions of the throat and mouth are sources of voiceless sounds. The opening or closing of a valve in the back of the mouth determines whether a sound is produced through the mouth or the nose. Each vowel and consonant of speech is a unique combination of tongue, lip, and lower jaw positioning. The pitch of the voice is determined by the tension of vocal folds in the larynx. The loudness of the voice depends on the air pressure from the lungs. The duration of each syllable of speech is determined by muscles of the chest. Some of these aspects of speech are seen in Figure 3–1.

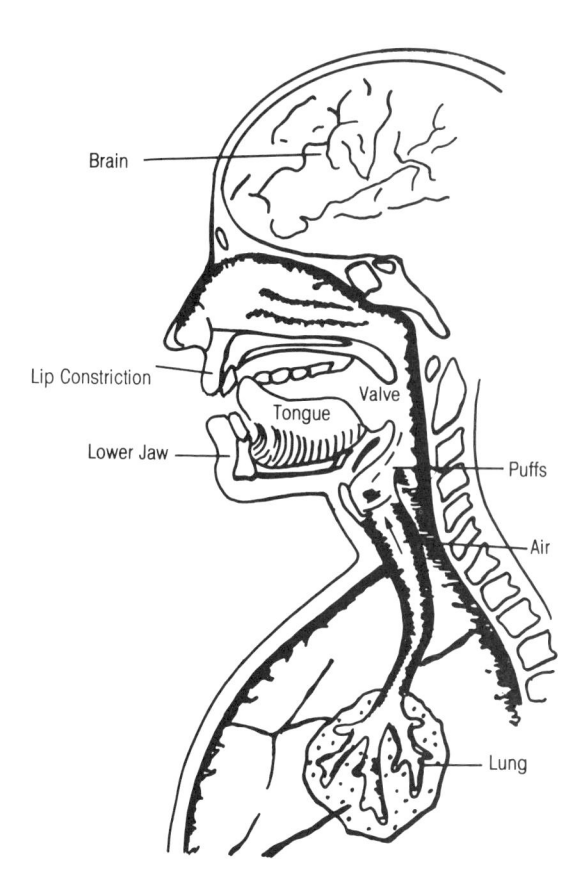

Figure 3-1. Parts and processes of the mechanism for producing speech sounds. From Potter, R., Kopp, K., and Green Kopp, H. (1966). *Visible speech* (p. 32). New York: Dover. Copyright 1966 by Dover Publications, Inc. Adapted by permission.

Speech Development and Hearing Loss

Speech normally develops during the first 7 to 8 years of the life of a person. During the first 6 months of life, children play with sounds and pitches if they can hear them. By 12 months of age, when words begin to emerge, children use many vowels and consonants. At 3 years, the sounds of speech of children are articulated well enough for their sentences to be understood by adults. By this time, all of the vowels and most of the consonants can be produced correctly. During the next 4 to 5 years, additional consonants are developed, and all consonants are produced in increasingly difficult combinations. The *s* in *spr* of the word *spring,* for example, is said correctly. During childhood the child is also learning to understand and say an increasingly larger vocabulary and more and more difficult sentences.

If hearing loss in both ears is present during childhood, speech does not develop as rapidly. A child who is deaf will not learn to speak at all unless given special instruction. A hard of hearing child will be delayed in speech development and will also require speech instruction. The vowels of hard of hearing children will tend to be produced correctly, but many of the consonants will be undeveloped or defective. Listening and language skills among hearing impaired children will be correspondingly undeveloped or incorrect. The lack of speech, listening, and language skills of these children will deter them from learning to read and write in school.

It is very important that parents and teachers do everything they can to help children with hearing losses learn to speak. Hearing impaired children initially need hearing aids to help them hear as well as possible. When children can hear, they can compare their own speech with the speech of others, comprehend the speech of others, and use their own speech meaningfully. Speech training is needed, however, in addition to hearing aids to assist hearing impaired children to form new speech habits.

Ordinarily, the greater the hearing loss, the longer a child requires to learn to listen and speak. For example, a child with a moderate loss may learn twice as fast as a child with a severe loss and eight times as fast as a child with a profound loss. This assumes that these three hypothetical children are wearing hearing aids. A speech acquisition program for a severely or profoundly hearing impaired child requires informed, systematic, and sustained effort over many years. The training required by children with less hearing loss corresponds to the number of speech skills they need to master.

A hearing impaired child should receive speech, listening, and language training as early in life as possible. One reason for beginning early is to prevent a child's cochlear or auditory nerve from deterioration due to lack of auditory stimulation. A second reason it to take advantage of the early years of life when language is most easily learned. A third reason is to not disturb the synchrony of sensory and motor development the child is undergoing without hearing. It is best that the child develop communication skills initially and not have to go through a more difficult and less successful rehabilitation process. When the hearing impaired child enters school with speech, listening, and language problems, it is very important that this child get sufficient help as quickly as possible.

Speech Sounds

The sounds of speech exceed in number the letters of the alphabet. There are 40 sounds and 26 letters. Of the 40 sounds, 15 are vowels and 25 consonants. Written symbols for the sounds are similar to but not exactly like the alphabet letters. The symbols for the sounds are called the International Phonetic Alphabet (IPA).

The speech-language pathologist, the educational audiologist, and the educator of the hearing impaired learn the IPA symbols and how each of the corresponding speech sounds are produced. They may also study the extent to which a particular hearing impaired child can hear each of these sounds with an appropriate hearing aid.

The classroom teacher can help one of these specialists with the speech remediation of a child by learning to identify correct and incorrect productions of the sounds of speech. The first learning step for the teacher is learning to identify each speech sound. This can be determined if the teacher can write down the IPA symbol for the sound when it is produced in a word or sentence. The second learning step for the teacher may be easier: The teacher simply has to listen and say whether a sound is produced correctly or incorrectly. Incorrect production is the omission, substitution, or distortion of a sound of speech. Table 3–1 shows a listing of IPA symbols and sample words in which sounds corresponding to the symbols occur.

The sounds of speech seldom appear alone. The basic unit of speech is the syllable. A syllable includes at least a vowel and usually one or more consonants. Each word includes one or more syllables. The words of Table 3–1 are single syllable words. Many words have two or more syllables. The word *Mississippi,* for example, has four syllables: mɪ—sɪ—sɪ—pɪ. A dictionary shows how words are broken into syllables. To teach children to pronounce words, teachers should know how to break polysyllabic words down into their component syllables. When words are said as fast as they appear in normal conversation, each syllable tends to begin with a consonant to make it easier to say words. It is correct to say words in this way, as exemplified in the word *Mississippi.*

Table 3-1. IPA Symbols and Words Including Speech Sounds

Symbol	Sample words
i	feet, sheep, teeth, bean, key, bee, beam, geese, cheese, deed, reel, cheek
ɪ	sit, pig, mitt, sing, whip, bib, fin, pin, hill, pick, ship, fish
e	vase, tape, cape, pail, lake, page, whale, gate, cane, veil, raise, baby
ɛ	egg, hedge jet, bear, ledge, men, net, leg, temple, shell, pear, bed
æ	cap, vat, bat, man, mat, badge, fang, fan, raft, jam, sash, patch
u	food, suit, shoe, root, hoop, zoo, tube, soup, noose, moon, ruler, boot
ʊ	foot, hood, bush, push, pulled, roof, woods, hook
o	coal, bow, ghost, cone, rope, fold, gopher, goat, phone, sore, toast, pole
ɔ	shawl, moth, hawk, ball, tongs, log, bought, doll
ɑ	arch, heart, sock, lock, jar, mop, large, car, garage, chop, knob, rock
ʌ	thumb, up, cup, gum, bug, gull, nut, bus, cuff, hub, tub, sun
aɪ	five, thigh, ice, light, hive, pile, tire, fire, line, vine, bison, bike
aʊ	down, hound, sow, house, tower, shout, scout, mouse
ɔɪ	foil, oink, boil, boy
ɪu	cute, few, huge, pew
f	foot, phone, file, feet, fire, fern, food, fish
θ	thigh, thong, thistle, thorn, think, thorax, thing, thimble
s	six, sash, sing, seal, sore, suit, sock, soup, surf, soap, safe, sack
ʃ	shade, shell, shoot, ship, shawl, shut, shine, shoe, shout, shove, shot, shirt
tʃ	cheek, chick, check, cheese, choke, church, chop, chair, chives, chimps, chapel, chief
h	hit, hedge, help, hook, hike, hound, hub, horse, hair, heart, hump, hawk
v	vest, vase, veil, vine, van, vault, view, valentine
ð	them, these, those, they, clothe, breathe, soothe, smooth
z	zipper, zoom, zone, zebra, bees, boys, pigs, eyes, beds, eggs, girls, dogs
dʒ	jam, juice, jewel, jail, jar, jump, juggle, jet, page, edge, hedge, bridge
p	peach, pen, pole, pig, pie, pearl, path, pan, push, pear, pipe
t	tail, taxi, tooth, teeth, tongue, tie, tape, tub, towel, table, turtle, television
k	king, cake, cane, key, comb, cone, curb, can, cup, kite, coat, car
b	bat, bag, bowl, bee, bug, bib, bird, ball, box, boat, bus, boot
d	door, dive, dome, dish, dam, dime, dark, deer, duck, down, dump, doll
g	gas, gun, gull, gum, geese, ghost, golf, gable, gag, girl
m	men, match, moth, moon, mice, muff, march, mouse, mop, mask, mug, milk
n	nail, neck, noose, net, knob, nuts, nine, knot, nerves, nibble, nag, knife
ŋ	sing, fang, bang, ring, tang, lung, rung, tongue
l	log, loaf, lad, lock, lake, light, line, leg, lamb, leash, latch, lip
r	reel, ring, raft, rib, root, road, reach, rake, rug, rag, round, rock
ɚ	chair, hair, door, car, fern, yard, thorn, barn, bark, lark, stork, fork
w	wig, wire, worm, web, weave, world, wasp, walk, wealth, woods, witch, wash
hw	whip, whelp, whirl, wheel
j	yacht, yam, yoke, yawn

Speech Considerations   45

Note also that the number of letters in a word often does not correspond to the number of sounds in a word. In the word *Mississippi,* there are 11 letters but only 8 sounds. The discrepancy between writing words and pronouncing them is also exemplified in the word *chauffeur,* which is spelled with 9 letters but pronounced with 4 sounds: ʃ of ɚ. An elementary or special education teacher needs considerable skill in phonetics, which is the study of the sounds of speech, to assist students to articulate speech sounds and pronounce words.

Often two or even three consonants appear together at the beginning or end of a syllable. An index of 133 vowels, single consonants, and double and triple consonants appears in Table 3–2. Notice that the sound /s/, for example, appears in 20 different s-combinations of this table. A child may

Table 3–2. Index of 133 Speech Articulation Targets

Program	Context	Program	Context	Program	Context	Program	Context
1	-i-	34	str-	67	-gz	100	bl-
2	-I-	35	spl-	68	-blz	101	br-
3	-e-	36	spr-	69	-ndz	102	-b
4	-ɛ-	37	-s	70	-plz	103	-bɚ
5	-æ-	38	-sn	71	-tṇz	104	-bḷ
6	-u-	39	-sp	72	-ʒ-,-ʒ-	105	d-
7	-ʊ-	40	-sk	73	dʒ	106	dr-
8	-o-	41	-st	74	-dʒ	107	-d
9	-ɔ-	42	-ks	75	p-	108	-ld
10	-ɑ-	43	-ts	76	pl-	109	-nd
11	-ʌ	44	-ps	77	pr-	110	-ṇd
12	-aɪ-	45	-stɚ	78	-p	111	-dɚ
13	-aʊ	46	-nts	79	-mp	112	-dḷ
14	-ɔɪ	47	ʃ-	80	-lp	113	-bd
15	-ɪu-	48	-ʃ	81	-pḷ	114	g-
16	f-	49	tʃ-	82	-mpḷ	115	gl-
17	fr-	50	-tʃ	83	t-	116	gr-
18	fl-	51	-ntʃ	84	tr-	117	-g
19	-f	52	h-	85	-t	118	-gd
20	-fs	53	v-	86	-nt	119	m-
21	-ft	54	-v	87	-tḷ	120	-m
22	-fts	55	-vz	88	-tṇ	121	n-
23	θ	56	-vd	89	-pt	122	-n
24	θr	57	ð-	90	-kt	123	-ŋ
25	-θ	58	-ð	91	k-	124	-ŋz
26	s-	49	z-	92	kl-	125	l-
27	sk-	60	-z	93	kr-	126	-l
28	sm-	61	-lz	94	kw-	127	r-
29	sn-	62	-mz	95	-k	128	-ɚ
30	sp-	63	-nz	96	-kɚ	129	-rn
31	st-	64	-zd	97	-kl	130	-rk
32	sl-	65	-bz	98	-ŋk	131	w-
33	sw-	66	-dz	99	b-	132	hw-
						133	j-

be able to say words with some of these s-combinations but should eventually be able to say words with all of them. Children who are 8 years of age normally can articulate all 133 sound targets.

Children need to learn to imitate these speech targets and to incorporate them into their spontaneous utterances. A child should be able to imitate each sound target by itself, in repeated syllables, in alternation with other syllables, and in syllable combinations at normal rate and with normal prosody. A speech-language pathologist or teacher of the hearing impaired follows a developmental order of difficulty in training children to say these targets.

Speech Programs

The child who is behind in developing speech skills also needs assistance in transferring imitated speech to spontaneous speech. Specific programs are included with the index of speech targets of Table 3–2. Each of 133 programs includes 4 to 12 picture, word, and sentence stimuli. The stimuli can be used to test or train a student. The stimuli for the first of the programs, which features the /i/ vowel target, are shown in Figure 3–2. Words within the language of the student are used. Each word may be trained under five conditions:

1. *Echoic.* The teacher looks at the printed word and says the word. The student has been instructed not to look at the stimulus page. The student listens to and looks at the teacher and repeats the word.
2. *Picture.* The teacher points to the picture. The student looks at it and says the word.
3. *Printed word.* The teacher points to the printed word. The student looks at it and says the word.
4. *Sentence completion.* The teacher looks at and says the incomplete sentence. The student listens to and looks at the teacher and says the complete sentence.
5. *Original sentence.* The teacher instructs the student to make up a sentence using the word. The student says an original sentence using the word.

Electronic Speech Aid

The sounds of speech can be visualized with an electronic speech aid called the Vocal Scope (Fig. 3–3). Both the teacher and the student can see unique radial patterns for each sound said carefully into the

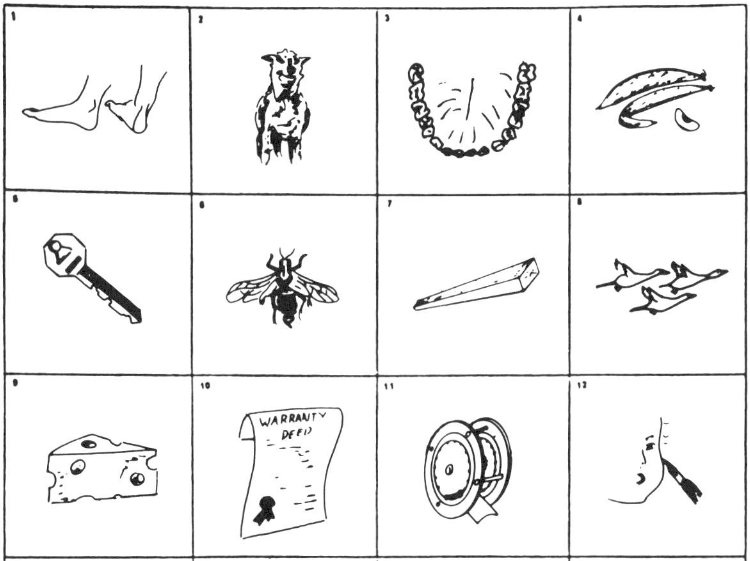

1	2	3	4
5	6	7	8
9	10	11	12

1 feet	2 sheep	3 teeth	4 bean
5 key	6 bee	7 beam	8 geese
9 cheese	10 deed	11 reel	12 cheek

1 Cover his ___.	2 Shear the ___.	3 Brush your ___.	4 Pick the ___.
5 Turn the ___.	6 Swat the ___.	7 Nail the ___.	8 Hunt the ___.
9 Slice the ___.	10 Sign the ___.	11 Wind the ___.	12 Touch her ___.

Figure 3-2. Twelve pictures and print stimuli for testing and training the / i / sound.

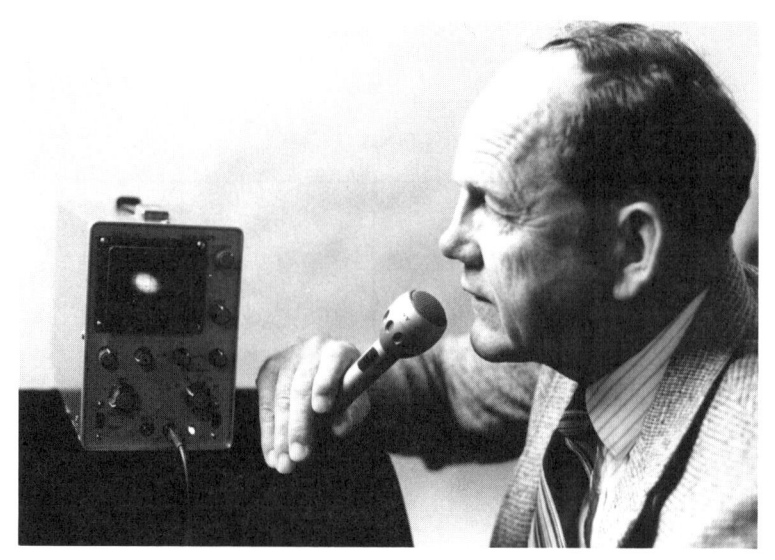

Figure 3-3. Vocal scope with radial pattern for the /s/ sound. From advertisement by F. Berg. Logan, UT: Amera Incorporated. Reprinted by permission.

microphone of the device. The /s/, for example, can be seen as many juxtapositioned circles. The teacher can say an /s/ and the student can try to match it.

The student can say any sound by itself, in a word, or in a sentence, and a visual pattern will appear on the screen. Only a minority of sounds are difficult to see; for example, /p/, which is very brief. When the student makes any sound, the teacher can listen to it and tell the student whether it is said right. The student will be able to associate visual patterns with correct and incorrect speech production.

Assisting the student to say a sound target correctly is the work of the speech-language pathologist or the teacher of the hearing impaired. Once a student produces a sound correctly, the regular teacher can assist in seeing that correct production is maintained, strengthened, and transferred into more words and sentences.

Visual patterns clarify what a person with normal hearing can hear. They may be even more important to a person who cannot hear a speech target or hear it completely. A speech aid like the Vocal Scope, however, should not be considered a substitute for a skilled speech specialist, a dedicated classroom teacher, a hearing aid, and appropriate speech programs. A speech aid is no more than a speech aid, and it has to be used appropriately to be effective.

Speech Screening and Parent Guidance

Speech-language pathologists in a school district have the responsibility to screen children for speech problems. Their screening efforts are concentrated on younger children so that problems can be identified early and speech training provided before bad speech habits are developed. Screening consists of listening to children say a sample of words or sentences, recording errors, and determining when children fail.

The stimuli and record form for a short speech check is shown in Table 3–3. Sixteen words are included. All of the 40 speech sounds are included at least once in the words. The pathologist says a word and the student repeats it. The pathologist draws a circle around the symbol for any sound that is omitted, substituted, or distorted. Comments on nonarticulatory speech problems are also recorded.

Most speech problems among children with and without hearing loss are articulation problems. The decision whether to provide a child with speech articulation assistance is based on a knowledge of ages at which speech sound targets normally develop. It is normal for kindergarten and first grade children to still have some speech articulation problems. When a young child also has a hearing loss in both ears, or has had bilateral hearing loss during the preschool years, that child is likely to be even less mature in speech articulation.

Some parents resist efforts to initiate speech training for their children. They do not want their children to be singled out as being different or needing special assistance. They may also believe that their children will master speech without assistance. Teachers can help parents realize (1) that it is very important to provide speech training for children and (2) the hearing loss complicates the persistence of a speech problem, unless speech training is provided.

Table 3–3. Speech Check

Words	Phonetic symbol	Word	Phonetic symbol
1. you	j u	9. ring	r ɪ ŋ
2. boy	b ɔ ɪ	10. wood	w ʊ d
3. show	ʃ o	11. goose	g u s
4. cow	k a ʊ	12. cage	k e dʒ
5. pie	p a ɪ	13. thumb	θ ʌ m
6. car	k a ɚ	14. cheese	tʃ ɪ z
7. earth	ɝ θ	15. feather	f ɛ ð ɚ
8. hat	h æ t	16. television	t ɛ l ə v ɪ ʒ ə n

Nonarticulation problems _____

Speech Problems

Precise speech is a highly desirable behavior in our culture. It is our main vehicle for expressing our thoughts and feelings to other people. A speech problem may interfer with communication, draw attention to itself, and cause its possessor to be maladjusted. Seven aspects of speech are described below.

Breath

A breath stream from the lungs powers the speech act. It sets the vocal folds into vibration for voiced sounds. It also moves through the throat and mouth, making possible the production of voiceless sounds. To speak, a person must be able to produce a steady and a pulsed (voiced) breath stream that coordinates with and basically supports production of the other aspects of speech.

Stress

The syllables of speech are normally produced with varying degrees of stress. The word *Mississippi* (mɪ sɪ sɪ pɪ) has most stress on the third syllable, next most on the first syllable, least on the second syllable, and next least on the last syllable. If this stress pattern is not used, communication may be adversely affected. A child with little or no hearing often has a problem in appropriately stressing syllables and words.

Voice

Most sounds of speech are voiced. This requires that the vocal folds of the larynx vibrate. The voice is pleasant when the vocal folds vibrate precisely. Vocal disorders occur when the folds are not coming together or separating on target. The quality of voice is largely determined by the precision of vocal fold vibration during speech. A breathy or husky voice, for example, is a problem to a child and needs early correction. A child with little or no hearing often has a voice problem.

Pitch

When a speech sound is vocalized it has a pitch. The pitch of the voice is determined by the rate at which the vocal folds vibrate. While saying a sentence, a person uses a range of pitches. People have different pitches because their vocal folds vary in length. Pitch, or vibrational rate, also depends upon vocal fold tension. Tension must be precisely adjusted or pitch will be inappropriate. Falsetto, or pitch above a person's normal pitch range, is an example of a profound pitch problem. The voices of children with little or no hearing are often fatigued from vocal fold tension heard as abnormal pitch.

Intonation

When a polysyllabic word, phrase, or sentence is being said, the pitch of a person's voice normally changes continually. This melody of speech is referred to as intonation. A sequence of pitch changes or intonation contour extends from each fully stressed syllable, for example, the third syllable of the word *Mississippi*. Meanings are often affected by changing intonation contours in sentences. Intonation is normally present in the vocalizations and speech of very young children. A child must be able to hear fine pitch differences to use normal intonation while speaking. A child with little or no hearing may have monotonous or uncontrolled speech intonation.

Nasality

During speech most speech energy naturally exits the mouth, and the three nasal consonants /m/, /n/, /ŋ/ through the nose. The positioning of a valve in the back of the mouth determines whether a speech sound is orally or nasally emitted. If the valve is closed, the sound comes through the mouth; if open, the sound comes through the nose. The ratio of oral sound to nasal sound is normally about 10:1. When valving is defective, sound that should be orally emitted spills into the nose and severely disturbs speech output. The vowels tend to be blurred, and the consonants lose their precision and crispness. Knowing whether the valve is shut or open depends on refined hearing. A child with a hearing loss often has speech that is too nasal. Too much nasality is called hypernasal; too little, hyponasal.

Articulation

Speech is also characterized by the forming and joining of the tongue, lips, and lower jaw to produce vowels and consonants in syllables, words, and sentences. This articulatory process is normally the last of the speech phenomena to mature. Many subskills have to be reached before this achievement occurs. Each vowel or consonant is a unique combination of the activity of the vocal folds, the valve in the back of the mouth, the constriction of the air stream in the mouth, and the place where articulation is occuring. Bilateral hearing loss complicates the mastery of speech sound articulation.

Teamwork

A child who is deaf or near deaf requires developmental speech training. All aspects of speech must be trained. The speech-language pathologist or educator of the hearing impaired, or both, will need to provide this training. Training must be systematic and sustained over many years. A child who is hard of hearing will have developed many speech skills naturally but still need considerable training. Each hearing impaired child will require careful evaluation to determine the extent of the speech problem and the point where training should begin. Developmental speech programs detail the training stages, steps, and subskills to develop. Strategies have been outlined, and training materials are commercially available. Regular classroom teachers and parents should work cooperatively with specialists in assisting children to master speech.

SUMMARY

Delayed or defective speech is highly prevalent among school children with bilateral hearing loss. Speech training must be provided for these children. Classroom teachers can assist speech-language pathologists and teachers of the hearing impaired to identify children with problems and to help them speak precisely. Regular teachers must learn to recognize the sounds of speech, to appropriately reinforce correct speech behavior, and to assist children to practice until the skills they have learned become automatic. Training guides, programmed materials, and electronic aids are available. Teachers should also encourage parents of the hearing impaired to support speech training that begins early in the lives of their children.

FURTHER READINGS

Daniel Ling's *Speech and the Hearing-Impaired Child* (Alexander Graham Bell Association for the Deaf, Washington, DC, 1976) is the basic reference for a developmental speech program for children with severe and profound bilateral hearing loss. Frederick Berg's *Speech Handbook* (Ear Products & Services, Smithfield, UT, 1986) includes speech articulation transfer programs and detailed information on the Vocal Scope. Skill in describing and recognizing the sounds of speech can be obtained through a *Home Study Phonetics Course* offered by Frederick Berg (Independent Study, UMC 50, Utah State University, Logan, UT 84322, (810)750-2131). The study material for this course is a handbook, a phonetics dictionary, an audio cassette, and Donald

Calvert's book *Descriptive Phonetics* (Thieme-Stratton, New York, 1980). More specialized speech considerations are detailed in the appendix of this chapter.

APPENDIX

How We Speak

Speech planning takes place in the brain before speech production occurs in the vocal tract. In the brain, meanings or ideas are coded into language and motor correlates before motor commands can be sent to the vocal tract to cause speech movements (MacNeilage, Studdert-Kennedy, and Lindblom, 1985). The language forms include semantic, syntactic, morphologic, and phonemic subforms. Semantic refers to the meaning of words, syntactic to sentence structure, morphologic to word structure, and phonemic to speech sound classes. We speak in a "hierarchy from phonemic feature, to phoneme, to syllable, to word, and to phrase and sentence" (Hirsh, 1985). Each phoneme produced includes several phonemic features. A feature of each vowel phoneme, for example, is absence of pressure buildup in the vocal tract, in distinction to each consonant phoneme, which has pressure buildup (Stevens, 1985). Stress and intonation features are also inherent in the syllables, words, phrases, and sentences of the speech act.

Speech can be meaningful or nonmeaningful. If meaningful, it is spoken language. If not, it is just a motor activity. In early speech development, the child babbles in nonmeaningful syllables. Later, the child speaks in words and sentences. As the child moves up the hierarchical ladder of speech from phonemes to long and complex sentences, speaking becomes more difficult. This difficulty is offset in part by hierarchical organization of speech units. Vowels, consonants, and syllables, for example, are incorporated into intonation and rhythmic patterns. Children use a self-organizing process to master the complicated interactive systems used to produce speech (Kent, 1985; Lauter, 1985).

To learn and use speech, information must be stored in the memory system of the brain (Bowe, 1985). The Atkinson and Shiffrin (1971) memory model provides one explanation for this process. Incoming stimuli are (1) entered in a sensory register; (2) quickly passed to short-term memory (STM), where they are coded and related to other information already in the system, and accepted or rejected; and (3) if accepted passed to long-term memory (LTM), where this information is available for future reference. When needed for speech, this information is passed back to short-term memory, where it can be rehearsed, and (4) tranferred to a response generator, which issues motor commands to speech muscles

(Atkinson and Shiffrin, 1971). This memory model appears in Figure 3-4.

Speech takes place over time. We speak at a rate of about 14 segments per second (MacNeilage et al., 1985). To say all possible speech sounds, syllables, words, and sentences intelligibly and fluently requires either preplanning (speech targets selected well in advance of speech movements), rapid sensory feedback with servo control, a cognitive schema that is highly responsive to various situational demands, or some combination of these (Bowe, 1985). There is evidence that the nerve cannot carry impulses fast enough to enable feedback to exercise moment-to-moment control over speech production. Ling (1976) has stated that feedback can only allow us to determine whether production has satisfied intention. Speech is functional when it is automatically or fluently produced. This occurs when we can concentrate on what we are saying rather than have to be concerned with how to produce speech (Stelmach and Hughes, 1985).

Speech feedback includes at least three types of loops: external sensory, internal sensory, and internal neural. When people speak, they hear what they say through air conducted and bone conducted sound. They also receive tactile feedback as their articulators (lips and tongue) lightly touch other surfaces, and proprioceptive feedback as their joints, tendons, and muscles of respiration, phonation, and articulation are stimulated (Warren, 1976). Feedback loops within the brain or central nervous system also seems to exist (Borden and Harris, 1984). The arrows of Boothroyd's (1985) speech model of Figure 3-5 schematizes

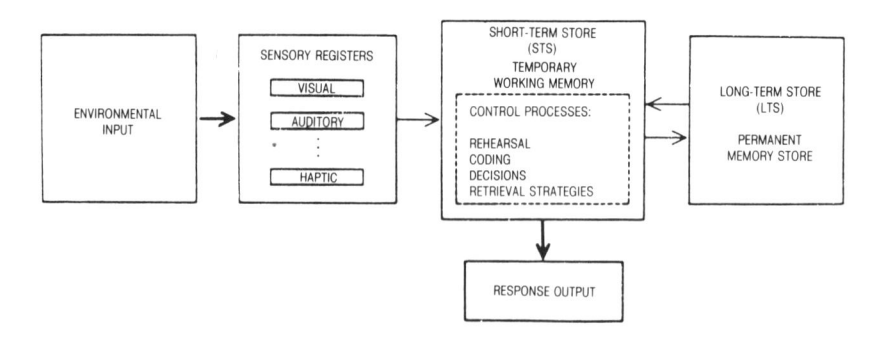

Figure 3-4. A model of how memory is involved in speech. From Atkinson, R., and Shiffrin, R. (1971). The control of short-term memory. *Scientific American, 225,* 82. Copyright 1971 by Scientific American, Inc. Reprinted by permission.

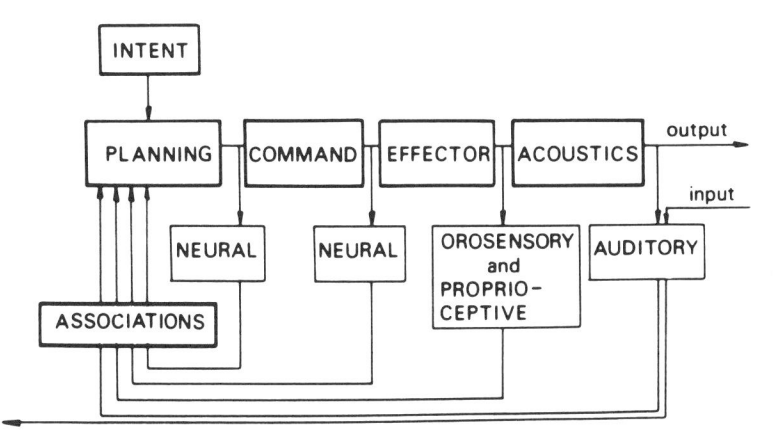

Figure 3-5. A model of external and internal feedback loops for speech planning and control. From Boothroyd, A. (1985). Residual hearing and the problem of carry-over in the speech of the deaf. In J. Lauder (Ed.), *Proceedings of the Conference on the Planning and Production of Speech in Normal and Hearing Impaired Individuals* (ASHA Reports 15, p. 8). Washington, DC: American Speech-Language-Hearing Association. Copyright 1985 by the American Speech-Language-Hearing Association. Reprinted by permission.

feedback loops. Children depend particularly on the auditory loop to learn speech. Hearing has a tremendously important role in the acquisition, generalization, and retention of motor speech skills, even in children with hearing losses in excess of 100 dB (Boothroyd, 1985).

The speaker has to breathe in a unique way while speaking (Fig. 3-6). In comparison with quiet breathing, more air is inspired, and more quickly, and expiration is much longer (Lauter, 1985). A word or sentence may be produced on the expiration part of one breath. The brain's control of speech respiration must be closely orchestrated with its control of speech articulation. The air pressure from the lungs must continously change in step with each successive phoneme produced.

Air pressure from the lungs must also be sufficient to assist with phonation or voice. During each cycle of phonation (vibration), pressure forces the vocal folds in the larynx to open and move outward. The outward movement continues because of momentum but is stopped and reversed by the elastic tension of the vocal folds. As the folds move inward and approach a closed position, the Bernoulli effect (sudden pressure drop due to narrow opening between folds) and causes them to close abruptly. Air pressure from the lungs and the elasticity of the

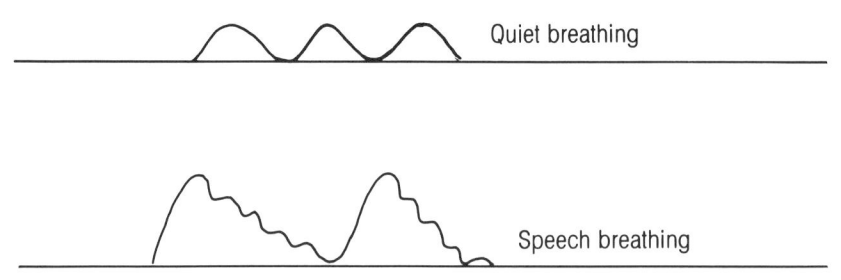

Figure 3-6. Comparison of amounts of inspiration–expiration cycles during quiet and speech breathing. From Borden, G., and Harris, K. (1984). *Speech science primer* (p. 73). Baltimore: Williams & Wilkins. Copyright 1984 by Williams & Wilkins. Adapted by permission.

closed folds causes this cycle to repeat itself (Pickett, 1980). The elasticity, tension, and mass of the folds determine the number of times this outward-inward cycle occurs per second. Adult men have the greatest vocal fold mass and therefore the lowest frequency (cycles per second) of vocal fold vibration. Adult women have less vocal fold mass, but they still have more than children, who have the highest frequency, or vocal pitch. If air pressure from the lungs is increased, the folds will open wider during each vibration cycle, producing a more intense voice (Borden and Harris, 1984).

"When we generate an utterance, we attempt to control the positions and movements of the articulatory structures and the respiratory system so as to achieve a certain pattern of acoustic goals or targets" (Stevens, 1985, p. 38). For an utterance to be understood by a listener, some aspects of these goals must be achieved with some precision while others can be approximated. Within a speaker-listener's brain is an inventory of more acoustic features than needed to produce or perceive the sounds and words of a language. To produce or perceive "bead" and "beet", for example, the /d/ is different from the /t/ on the basis of (1) presence or absence of voicing, (2) duration of the preceding vowel, and (3) intensity and duration of the burst of noise as these words are released or terminated. The additional features beyond what is minimally needed to differentiate these words are called redundant features. Redundancy in an utterance counteracts the effect of factors that make listening more difficult, such as room noise. Speech is also more understandable when it is slowed down, allowing the listener additional time to decode the units of an utterance (Stevens, 1985).

Hearing Loss and Speech

Children with congenital or early hearing loss have speech problems. If some hearing loss in both ears is involved, there is delay in speech development unless special stimulation is provided. If more serious hearing loss exists, speech is permanently defective unless special training is provided. Children with bilateral hearing loss exceeding 100 dB do not develop all vocal, prosodic, and articulatory skills and speak unnaturally unless they receive informed, systematic, and sustained training (Ling, 1976). Educators should be concerned when there is delayed, defective, or unnatural speech among children because of the adverse communicative and socioemotional effects of these deficits. The relationship between hearing loss and speech production is explained more fully in the professional literature (Berg, 1976; Boothroyd, 1982; Calvert and Silverman, 1975; Erber, 1982; Ling 1976).

Notwithstanding the deleterious effect of hearing loss upon speech, even children with 100 dB loss can perceive more vocal, prosodic, and articulatory features through residual hearing than through lipreading (Ling, 1976). The role of a hearing aid in making this possible will be described in Chapter 6. The remaining hearing provides deep speech cues from the vocal tract, whereas lipreading provides only surface speech cues. Vocal and prosodic features of speech are produced deep in the vocal tract and can be at least partially perceived through residual hearing. Articulatory cues also are mainly deep cues. For example, tongue movements determine speech articulation more than lip or jaw movements. The tongue movements are largely hidden from view (Boothroyd, 1982).

Table 3–4 suggests the relative contributions of hearing and lipreading cues to speech perception by a child with an average of 100 dB hearing loss and ability to hear only low frequencies of speech (Berg, 1976; Boothroyd, 1985). Separate comparisions for perception of stress patterns, voice-voiceless distinction, oral-nasal distinction, restriction (manner) of articulation, and place of articulation are shown. Figure 3–7 shows these vocal, prosodic, and articulatory features within the vocal tract (Berg, 1976). A similar comparison of the relationship of decibel loss and perception of speech features has been made by Boothroyd (1985), based on his experience with preschool children at the Clarke School for the Deaf. He notes that perception of place of articulation begins to be adversely affected when hearing loss exceeds 50 dB, and vowel height when loss is more than 100 dB. While at the Central Institute for the Deaf, Erber (1982) made similar observations.

Children with 110 to 120 dB hearing losses will not auditorily per-

Table 3-4. Possible Perception of Speech Features by a Child with a 100 dB Bilateral Loss

Speech feature	Hearing	Lipreading
1. Stress patterns	Mainly perceived	Not perceived
2. Pitch patterns	Broad changes perceived	Not perceived
3. Voiced-voiceless	Perceived if syllable stressed	Not perceived
4. Oral-nasal	Perceived if syllable stressed	Not perceived
5. Unrestricted, restricted, or momentarily stopped	Perceived if syllable stressed	Perceived if syllable stressed
6. Tongue position primarily; lip and jaw position and other points of articulation	Mainly perceived if syllable stressed	Partially perceived if syllable stressed

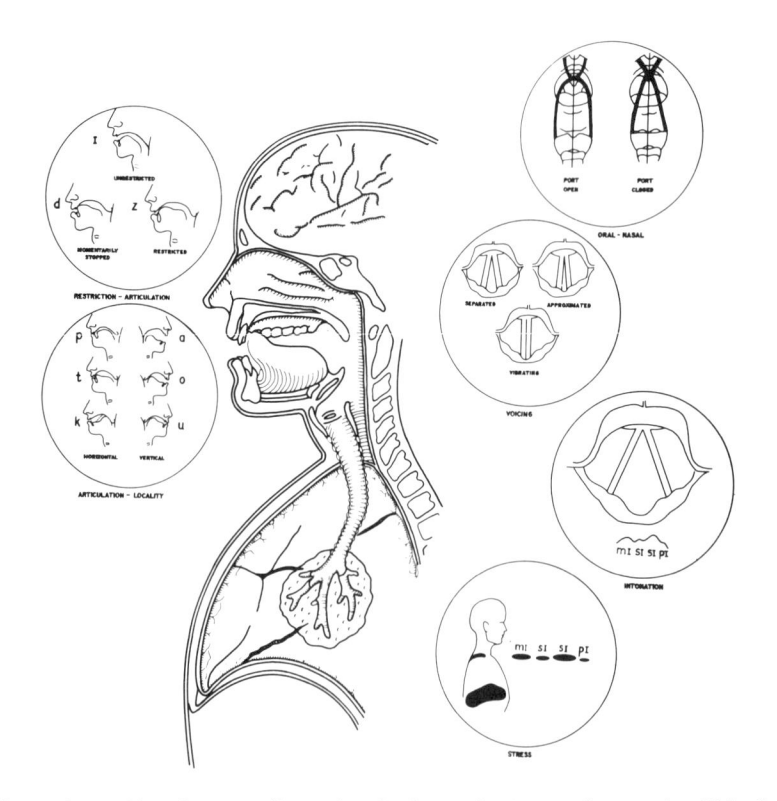

Figure 3-7. Vocal, prosodic and articulatory features of speech within the vocal tract. From Potter, R., Kopp, G., and Green Kopp, H. (1966). *Visible speech* (p. 32). New York: Dover. Copyright 1966 by Dover Publication, Inc. Adapted by permission.

ceive speech well. Children with 90 dB losses or less will perceive speech better. There are always exceptions to this generalization. Only testing and training will determine how well a particular child perceives or can learn to perceive speech features. In this connection, it is of interest that most children in schools for the deaf can detect low and middle speech frequency energies. When children can not only detect these frequencies but have learned to use speech cues within this frequency band to recognize words and sentences, they function as hard of hearing rather than deaf children (Berg, 1976; Wedenberg and Wedenberg, 1970).

Ling (1976) advocates the use of hearing, vision, and touch in a developmental speech program for a hearing impaired child. Initially, breathing, vocal, and prosodic skills are of concern, and then the many articulation skills. With a hard of hearing child, training ordinarily begins with consonant articulation skills (Berg, 1976).

Speech must be developed at both imitative (phonetic) and spontaneous (phonologic) levels (Ling, 1976). The levels and skills required are (1) producing speech patterns, (2) auditorily differentiating one's own speech patterns, (3) listening to others' speech patterns and comparing them with one's own speech patterns, (4) comprehending the meaning of others' speech, and (5) using one's own speech meaningfully. Phonetic drill is used to compensate for previously missed prelinguistic utterance practice, basic to normal spoken language acquisition. Phonologic activities are used to transfer imitative speech skills into meaningful utterances.

Language Training

Children talk more effectively if they are competent in language as well as in speech. Hearing impaired children typically are deficient in both language and speech. Therefore, language training is also given to hearing impaired children by speech-language pathologists and educators of the hearing impaired. The functional and pragmatic use of language is emphasized in current language programming. Simon (1980), for example, has developed a comprehensive language program for school children based on competent versus incompetent communicative skills (Fig. 3–8).

The Simon program may be divided into three developmental levels: (1) emerging language, (2) syntactical-morphological development, and (3) form, style, and functional expansion. Students learn how to formulate effective messages that are listening oriented, coherent, fluent, and composed of adult grammar. A functional-pragmatic language test is initially given a student. The test results suggest which communication skills the child needs to develop. Short-term criterion based objectives are then written, and language materials are selected.

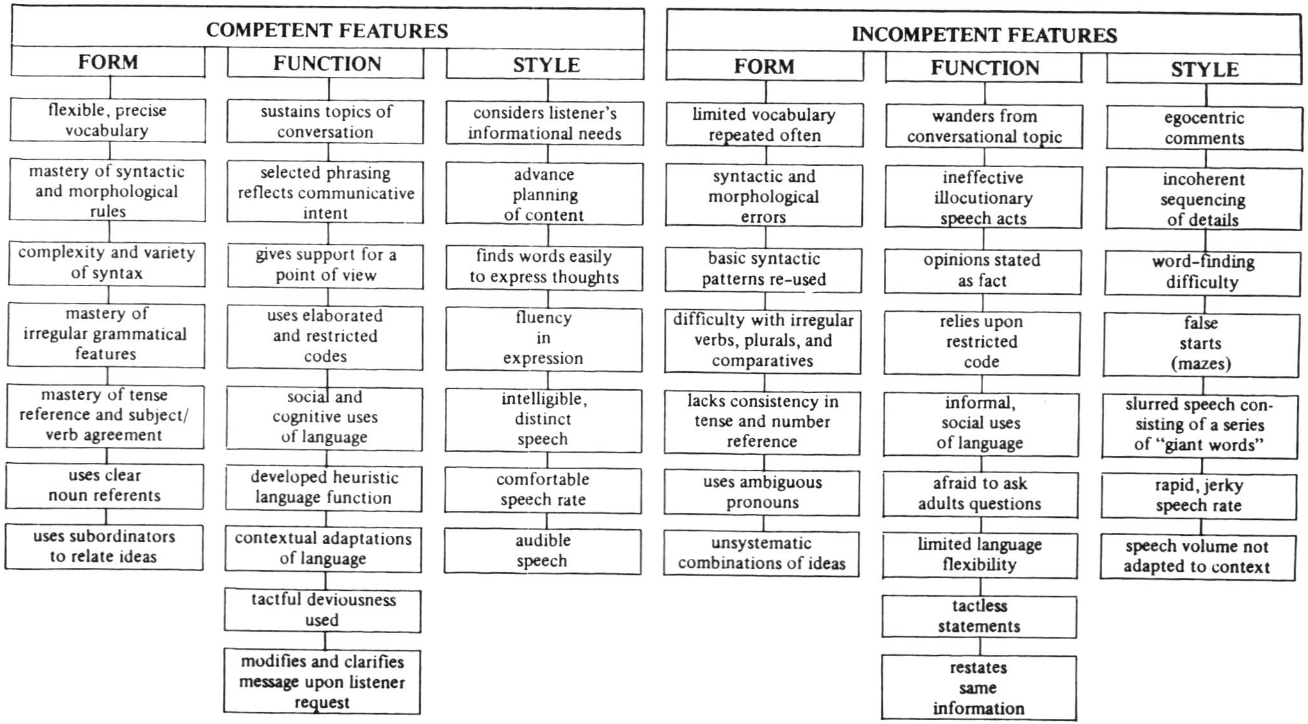

COMPETENT FEATURES

FORM	FUNCTION	STYLE
flexible, precise vocabulary	sustains topics of conversation	considers listener's informational needs
mastery of syntactic and morphological rules	selected phrasing reflects communicative intent	advance planning of content
complexity and variety of syntax	gives support for a point of view	finds words easily to express thoughts
mastery of irregular grammatical features	uses elaborated and restricted codes	fluency in expression
mastery of tense reference and subject/verb agreement	social and cognitive uses of language	intelligible, distinct speech
uses clear noun referents	developed heuristic language function	comfortable speech rate
uses subordinators to relate ideas	contextual adaptations of language	audible speech
	tactful deviousness used	
	modifies and clarifies message upon listener request	

INCOMPETENT FEATURES

FORM	FUNCTION	STYLE
limited vocabulary repeated often	wanders from conversational topic	egocentric comments
syntactic and morphological errors	ineffective illocutionary speech acts	incoherent sequencing of details
basic syntactic patterns re-used	opinions stated as fact	word-finding difficulty
difficulty with irregular verbs, plurals, and comparatives	relies upon restricted code	false starts (mazes)
lacks consistency in tense and number reference	informal, social uses of language	slurred speech consisting of a series of "giant words"
uses ambiguous pronouns	afraid to ask adults questions	rapid, jerky speech rate
unsystematic combinations of ideas	limited language flexibility	speech volume not adapted to context
	tactless statements	
	restates same information	

Figure 3–8. Model of expressive communicative competence. From Simon C. (1980). *Communicative competence: a functional-pragmatic language program* (p. xiii). Tucson: Communication Skill Builders. Copyright 1980 by Communication Skill Builders. Reprinted by permission.

Simon's test and training procedures, together with instructional materials, are included in a storage box available from Communication Skill Builders (Tucson, Arizona). A theoretical monograph, a teaching manual, filmstrips, a photo-diagram book, stimulus cards, and spinners are included. The manual describes the communicative tasks that can be programmed with the stimulus materials. Language specialists supplement the Simon materials with other commercially available materials and with those they develop themselves.

The correlation between speech training and language training is exemplified in Simon's program when teaching the third person singular -s marker. In speech, the word-final /s/ target has been taught. A sequential story print out from Simon's photo-diagram book is used. The student is asked to look at the sequence of actions and then tell about the event. The student is also reminded to remember the special words. An example of procedure and materials appear below.

> Look at the sequence of the lady doing the laundry. Say to the student "Each Saturday she does the laundry. These are the things she does during this job. Tell me what she does. Remember the buzz at the end of the action words. Okay, tell me what she does each Saturday."
>
> Student: "She gets the clothes. She turns on the washer. She puts in soap. She puts in the clothes. She puts them in the dryer. She takes them out. She folds them."
>
> Teacher: "Good! You remembered to put the buzz on each action word. She gets the clothes. She turns on the washer. She puts in the soap. She puts them in the dryer. She takes them out. She folds them."

Chapter 4

Listening Considerations

CASE STUDY

JA is a 13 year old junior high school student. Until recently he has had top grades in school. Last month the quality of his school work dropped, and he complained he could not hear. The school principal recommended that his parents take him to an audiologist for hearing testing and to a otologist for hearing diagnosis. Both the audiologist and otologist are located in a hearing center in a nearby community. JA's parents have been very concerned about his problem and promptly phoned the hearing center for appointments with the audiologist and otologist.

The audiologist forwarded to the school a copy of a report on JA that included his audiograms. The report indicates JA has a 60 dB sensorineural hearing loss in each ear, with greatest impairment for high frequency sounds. It also recommends that JA be fitted with a hearing aid. The audiologist states that the aid will not bring back normal hearing but that it should help him.

The audiologist has consulted with the otologist who reports that JA's hearing loss is permanent and cannot be medically or surgically helped. The otologist also recommends a hearing aid. In interviewing the parents, the otologist has discovered that the mother's side of JA's family has a history of inherited "deafness" that usually occurs after birth. This seems to be the cause of JA's hearing loss.

Yesterday JA showed up at school with a hearing aid. JA says it helps him hear better but not as well as originally. A district speech-language pathologist has been given primary responsibility by the district special education director to see that JA's special needs are met. The school principal has assigned a student study team to develop an Individualized Educational Plan (IEP) for JA. Members of the team include his parents, the principal, his teachers, the special education director, the speech-language pathologist, and JA.

Of primary concern is understanding the impact of JA's hearing loss and hearing aid upon his listening and learning skills in school. Further testing by the audiologist has revealed that JA cannot consistently repeat back words and sentences, even when using his hearing aid. When sound is made comfortably loud for him, he repeats only 50 percent of lists of words and sentences presented to him. It is not a problem of his not knowing how to speak precisely or of no longer remembering what the words and sentence mean. He just does not discriminate sounds as well as he used to, even when he is in a quiet and nonreverberant room. If he did not have this discrimination problem, with his hearing aid he would be able to repeat 100 percent of the words or sentences, or nearly so, in a quiet room and at close distance.

An identified area of need for an IEP, therefore, is improvement in listening performance. A long-term goal and short-term instructional objectives should be directed at improving JA's listening performance. It is impossible to predict whether JA's listening performance will improve, and if so, by just what amount. Listening training, however, should be provided, to bring him as close to his listening potential as possible. Whereas his listening performance under ideal conditions is 50 percent, his listening potential may be greater than 50 percent and even reach 100 percent.

If JA's listening performance could be improved, he should do better in school. As it is, he misunderstands a great deal of classroom instruction and direction. He also has a very difficult time in conversing with his parents and peers. Of course, he does better when he can lipread or face the talker, but even then he does not catch everything that is said.

When JA does not wear his hearing aid, his listening performance is almost zero unless he is lipreading or the speaker gets close to him and talks very loudly. Another identified need is for JA's teachers and parents to understand the effects of various degrees of hearing loss upon listening performance. JA's hearing loss varies according to whether he is using his aid, how much the aid's volume control is turned up, and the distance between himself and the person speaking.

BASICS OF LISTENING

Importance

The culture in which people live rewards a good listener and discriminates against a poor one. Those who perceive speech effectively realize personal, social, and economic benefits that a poor listener does not. A continuing need exists to upgrade listening skills among people. Modern technologies such as tape recorders and personal computers can be utilized to assist in the accomplishment of this task. School should be a place where listening skills are taught and encouraged.

Definitions and Processes

Listening may be defined as detection, discrimination, recognition, or comprehension of speech through audition, vision, or both in combination. Speech detection is awareness of the presence of speech sounds, words, or sentences. Speech discrimination is distinguishing one speech sound, word, or sentence from one or more other speech sounds, words, or sentences. Speech recognition is being able to repeat a sound, word, or sentence. Speech comprehension is understanding concepts of spoken language or messages.

Audition refers to hearing and the ears. Vision refers to sight and the eyes. Sometimes people listen to speech with their ears, sometimes with their eyes (lipreading or speechreading), and sometimes with both ears and eyes. Over the telephone, the ears normally provide clear sensory input. Using the eyes or lipreading only does not ordinarily provide sufficient information for understanding speech. In school, teachers and children use both their ears and their eyes when they are unsure of what is being said.

People listen to sound in general, not just to speech, with their ears. Sound must be detected before it can be discriminated from other sounds, recognized as being distinct from all other sounds, and comprehended (Fig. 4–1). Sometimes it is as important to listen to environmental sounds like a telephone or a doorbell ring as it is to catch a particular word.

People selectively attend to certain sounds and sights and reject others. The stimuli persons should attend to are referred to as "signals." The stimuli persons should reject are called "noise." During classroom instruction, for example, the teacher's voice is the signal, and other children talking out of turn are noise.

66   Facilitating Classroom Listening

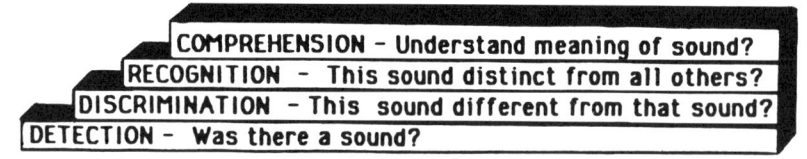

```
COMPREHENSION - Understand meaning of sound?
RECOGNITION   - This sound distinct from all others?
DISCRIMINATION - This sound different from that sound?
DETECTION - Was there a sound?
```

Figure 4-1. Listening processing levels from detection to comprehension of sound.

Sound localization, determining where sound originates, also contributes to general listening effectiveness. Having two ears makes it possible, but learning is also involved. If people can localize sound, they do not have to continually scan their environment visually to keep track of where things are happening.

Listening Development

Children develop listening skills before and during the time they are in school. During infancy, they learn basic listening skills such as attending, localizing, and discriminating sounds. During the preschool years, when children develop considerable speech and language, they learn to recognize and comprehend an increasing store of words, sentences, and environmental events. In elementary and secondary school, listening activities involve increasingly difficult memory and comprehension tasks.

Hearing impaired children need special stimulation and training in the development of listening skills. Listening, language, and speech training should begin as early as possible in life. A listening attitude needs to be trained because hearing impaired children naturally learn to rely on vision. A hierarchy of listening and speech tasks must be learned before a hearing impaired child can be expected to succeed in regular school.

Individual daily tutoring in listening and speech must be given to young school children with severe and profound bilateral hearing losses. The listening and speech targets of the tutoring sessions are then included in classroom and home learning experiences. Children are trained to recognize and repeat syllables, words, and sentences. They learn to listen and tell simple stories, to answer questions about interesting happenings, and to sing with appropriate melody. An example of a song sung with natural pitch pattern may be

> Hopping, hopping, hopping, hopping,
> Goes the bunny down the trail.
> Hopping, hopping, hopping, hopping,
> Wiggling his little tail.

Young hearing-impaired children with less severe hearing impairment can be stimulated or trained to develop basic listening, language, and speech skills more naturally. Of course they also need to be fitted with hearing aids. Parents must talk to them while they are involved in enjoyable activities. Rules for talking are followed, such as these: talk about here and now, talk about the obvious. At times, the parents talk for the child and put the child's feelings into words.

In school, a special listening program enhances the basic development of speech discrimination, recognition, and comprehension skills. An example of a task from each stage of a five stage training program appears here.

Prosodic discrimination: chair, table, bicycle, television.
Sentence recognition: Write your last name on the paper.
Word recognition: swim, stun, fret, bikes.
Phonetic discrimination: beef, bit, bait, bet, bat.
Message comprehension: A red fox lives in the meadow near the woods. It hunts food at night. It eats meadow mice. It likes to steal chickens.

A child begins this program at the point where he is having difficulty. This is determined from an accompanying listening test. Training may be given through audition, vision, or combined audition-vision.

The elementary and secondary school curricula provide extensive opportunity for practice in attending to and localizing sound, and in discriminating, recognizing, and comprehending words, sentences, and messages. Listening is involved in classroom instruction in language arts, social studies, mathematics, natural sciences, and related curricular areas. Conversation, story telling, laboratory experiences, and many other school experiences can be used by teachers to enhance listening.

Detection Information

Basic to listening is detecting the presence of as many of the sounds of speech as possible. The vowels and consonants vary in intensity from the /ə/, which is the faintest sound, to /ɑ/, which is one of the most intense sounds. A normal hearing child may hear all of the 40 speech sounds, whereas a hard of hearing child may only hear some of them, and a completely deaf child, none of them, even with a hearing aid. Hearing aids enable hard of hearing children to hear more of the sounds of speech than they ordinarily do, but not necessarily all of them. The number of sounds hard of hearing children can hear with hearing aids depends on their hearing losses.

Hearing tests are administered to children to determine whether they have hearing losses that might prevent them from hearing the

68 Facilitating Classroom Listening

sounds of speech. Pure tones rather than speech sounds are used as test stimuli. A pure tone has the advantage of being a single frequency or vibration rate. In contrast, each consonant or vowel includes many simultaneously produced frequencies or vibration rates.

An audiometer is used to generate the pure tones that are used in hearing testing (Fig. 4–2). Pure tones with frequencies of 125, 250, 500, 1000, 2000, 4000, and 8000 vibrations per second (Hz) are used as test stimuli. These frequencies are representative of the low, middle, and high frequencies of the sounds of speech. Each of these pure tones is an octave apart in frequency, beginning with a tone that is like the fundamental frequency of the male adult voice and ending with a tone that is included in the highest frequency consonant sound, the /s/.

Each of the 125, 250, 500, 1000, 2000, 4000, and 8000 Hz pure tones of the audiometer can be varied in intensity. The faintest intensity for each pure tone can be heard only if a person has very sensitive hearing. The greatest intensity for each pure tone is uncomfortably loud. The range of intensity is expressed in decibel (dB) values. When a pure tone is presented so that normal hearing people can just barely hear it, its value of 0 dB. When it is presented at its highest intensity, its

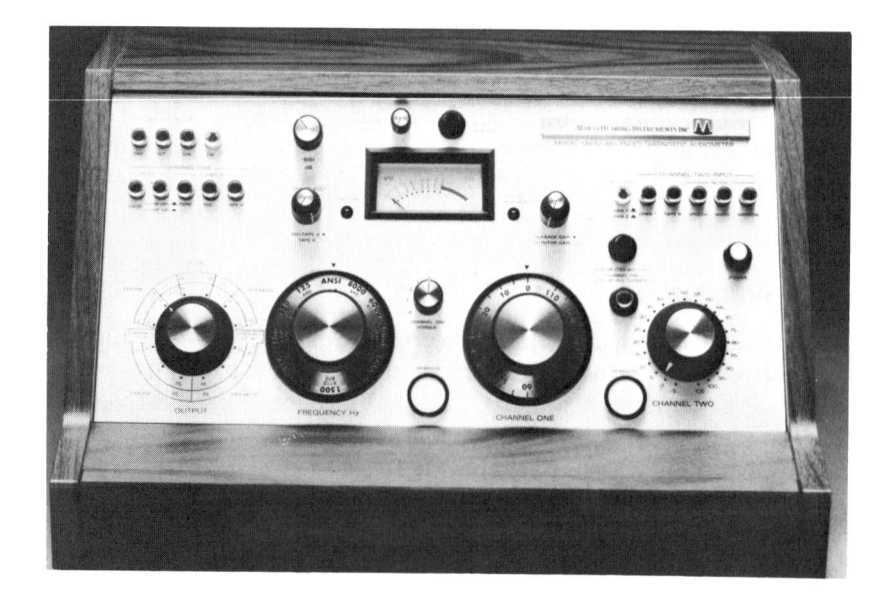

Figure 4–2. An audiometer. From MAICO Model MA32 diagnostic audiometer advertisement. Minneapolis: Maico Hearing Instruments Co. Reprinted by permission.

value may be 100 dB. A tone of 100 dB is 10 billion times more intense than a tone of 0 dB.

During hearing testing, audiologists determine how much hearing loss exists at each pure tone frequency in each ear of the person being tested. The pure tones are presented through earphones. Audiometer switches enable the audiologist to turn the power on, present different frequencies, and deliver the pure tones into the right ear or the left ear. Another audiometer control allows a tone to be varied in intensity from −10 dB to as high as 80 to 110 dB. The sound intensity is either increased or decreased until a sound threshold for a particular frequency is determined. The threshold is where the person being tested begins to detect the presence of the pure tone. This procedure is repeated for each pure tone and each ear.

Audiologists record detection thresholds on audiogram forms (Fig. 4–3). Circles are used to record thresholds in the right ear. Crosses are used to record thresholds in the left ear. If the intensity control on the audiometer has to be increased to 15 dB or more before a threshold is reached, this is outside the normal range of hearing and indicative of a pathologic condition and hearing loss. This is particularly true for test frequencies of 500, 1000, and 2000 Hz, where speech information is especially concentrated. The average hearing loss for each ear is calculated by adding the dB values of the detection thresholds for each of these frequencies, and dividing the sum by three. If the thresholds for 500, 1000, and 2000 Hz for the right ear, for example, were 20, 25, and 30 dB, respectively, the sum would be 75 dB and the average hearing loss 25 dB. If the corresponding thresholds for the left ear were 25, 30, and 35 dB, the average hearing loss would be 30 dB. The average hearing loss for each ear should be recorded.

Audiograms indicate degree of hearing loss. The more the audiogram is depressed, the worse the sound detection. The effects of three degrees of detection loss in one ear and in both ears are predicted here. It is assumed that the student is listening in a typical classroom environment 12 feet from the sound source (classroom teacher) and without a hearing aid or FM amplification equipment.

- Slight unilateral, 11 to 25 dB. Only loud speech sounds from impaired-ear side of head tend to be detected.
- Mild unilateral, 26 to 45 dB. Only loud speech sounds from impaired-ear side of head are detected.
- Moderate to profound unilateral, 46 to 100+ dB. No speech sounds from impaired-ear side of head tend to be detected.
- Slight bilateral, 11 to 25 dB. Only loud speech sounds from either side of head tend to be detected.
- Mild bilateral, 26 to 45 dB. Only loud speech sounds from either side of head are detected.
- Moderate to profound bilateral, 46 to 100 dB. No speech sounds from either side of head are detected.

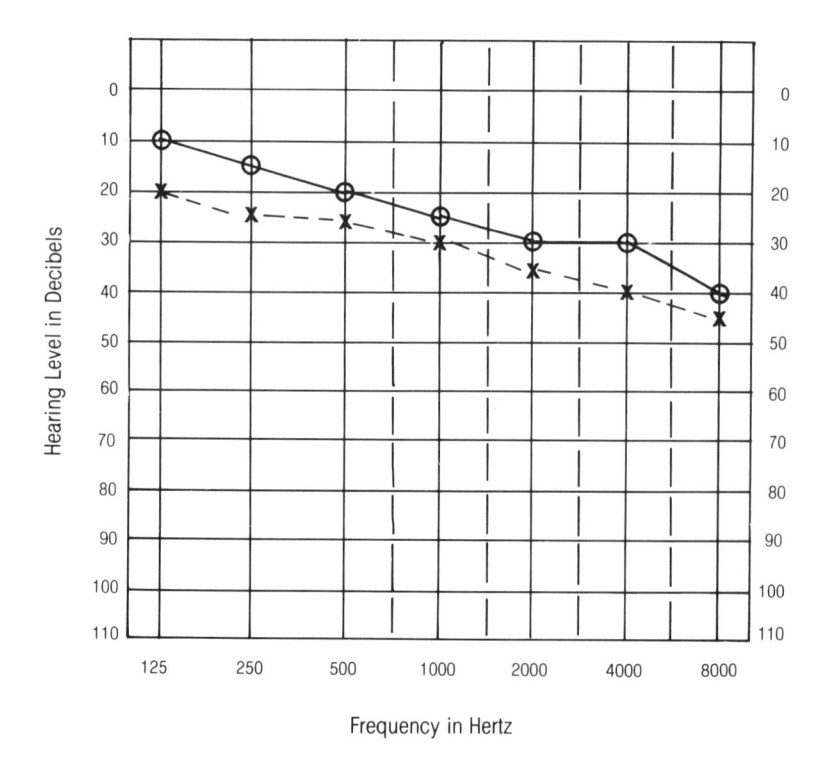

Figure 4-3. Audiogram form and recorded detection thresholds for the right ear and left ear of a hearing impaired person.

Understanding Speech

Speech sounds must be above a person's detection threshold in at least one ear before they can be heard. As the intensity of sound is gradually increased above threshold, a higher and higher percentage of speech sounds can be identified, resulting in a higher percentage of words recognized. With a 30 to 40 dB increase from a person's detection threshold, a person's word recognition percentage may increase from 0 percent to 100 percent, if that person has normal hearing or a conductive hearing loss. If a person has a sensorineural hearing loss or a pathologic condition of the auditory nerve, word recognition percentage does not usually reach 100 percent, no matter how intensely words are presented.

Listening training can increase the percentage of speech sounds and words recognized by a person with a sensorineural hearing loss, provided all speech sounds are loud enough to be comfortably detected. The extreme example is the near deaf person whose speech sound and word recognition scores improved from 0 to 100 percent after 4 hours of training. Not all the frequencies of a speech sound need to be heard by a person receiving listening training before the person can recognize that speech sound. Only a few unique sound cues may need to be heard for sound or word recognition to be learned.

It is extremely important that a hearing impaired person be able to detect and learn to recognize as many sounds of speech as possible. A combination of detection and recognition of sound is the basis for learning speech and spoken language and communicating with others through speech. It is important that listening training be given as needed.

To be detected and recognized, speech sounds should be comfortably loud. If speech is too soft, it cannot be detected. If speech is too loud, it will sound distorted and be uncomfortable for the listener. During audiometric testing, detection thresholds should be obtained not only for each test frequency but also for discomfort thresholds. This can be done for each frequency by increasing the intensity control of the audiometer to the point where a person reports the sound is becoming too loud. Ordinarily this needs to be done only at 500, 1000, and 2000 Hz for each ear. Each discomfort threshold can be marked with a *D* on the audiogram form.

The decibel difference between a person's detection threshold and his or her discomfort threshold is the person's listening range. If the detection threshold is 60 dB, for example, and the discomfort threshold is 100 dB, the listening range is 40 dB. This range is sufficient for listening, since the dB difference between the faintest and the most intense speech sounds is 30 dB. If the faintest speech sounds are presented at least 10 dB above a person's detection threshold, the most intense speech sounds will be 40 dB above that person's threshold. This ordinarily works well for hard of hearing children in regular classes.

Children with very severe hearing impairment often have a listening range of less than 30 dB. A special hearing aid that compresses speech is often helpful for these children. With this type of aid, the dB difference between faint and loud speech sounds may now be as little as 10 dB. Often this compensation enables a hearing impaired child to listen effectively when faint speech sounds are 10 dB above that child's detection thresholds.

Hearing Screening

In each class of school there are students who do not listen effectively. Some have detection problems, others recognition problems, and still others cognitive and memory problems. Pathologic conditions of the ear and presumed mininal brain damage are causative agents. In certain instances, the classroom teacher may not be aware that a child has a listening problem and may mistake it for a behavior problem.

The main cause of listening problems among students in school is hearing loss. Often the hearing loss is conductive; many students also have sensorineural hearing loss. In Chapter 2, the impedance meter and the acoustic otoscope were described as instruments for identifying children with conductive hearing loss. In this chapter, the audiometer and earphones have been described for obtaining detection thresholds of conductive, sensorineural, or mixed hearing loss.

An audiometer and earphones are also used for hearing screening. A pure tone sweep check is quickly administered to a child by an audiologist, speech-language pathologist, or school nurse. The four frequencies 500, 1000, 2000, and 4000 Hz are screening test tones. These tones represent the low, middle, and high frequencies of speech sounds. At each frequency, the intensity control is set at 20 dB above the normal detection threshold. Students who can detect 20 dB pure tones through earphones can detect faint speech sounds at close distances, unless the testing environment is noisy. It is best when hearing screening can be conducted in an audiometric test booth (Fig. 4–4), which is specially constructed to keep out interfering noise.

A new handheld hearing screening device, called an audioscope, can be used in place of the larger audiometer. A classroom teacher may be trained to use this device under the supervision of a specialist. The screening procedure for one ear takes as little as 15 seconds. A start button activates an automatic screening cycle. Within a cycle the 500, 1000, 2000, and 4000 Hz tones are presented at 20 dB. The tester watches the listener to see that he or she responds each time the tone is presented. A light below each frequency indication goes on each time a tone is presented. The start button can be pushed again to repeat a test cycle. Power is provided by a rechargeable battery. Figure 4–5 shows and lists procedures for screening with an audioscope.

Audiologists, or speech-language pathologists supervised by audiologists, should obtain audiograms on children who do not pass a hearing screen. The appendix of this chapter provides further information on hearing testing and audiograms. Audiograms for each ear will reveal the extent to which the sounds of speech can be detected by the child (Fig. 4–6).

Simulating Hearing Loss

The effect of increasing the sound detection loss upon listening can be simulated with a tape recording. Begin by listening to a message that has not been reduced in intensity. Continue to listen with the intensity

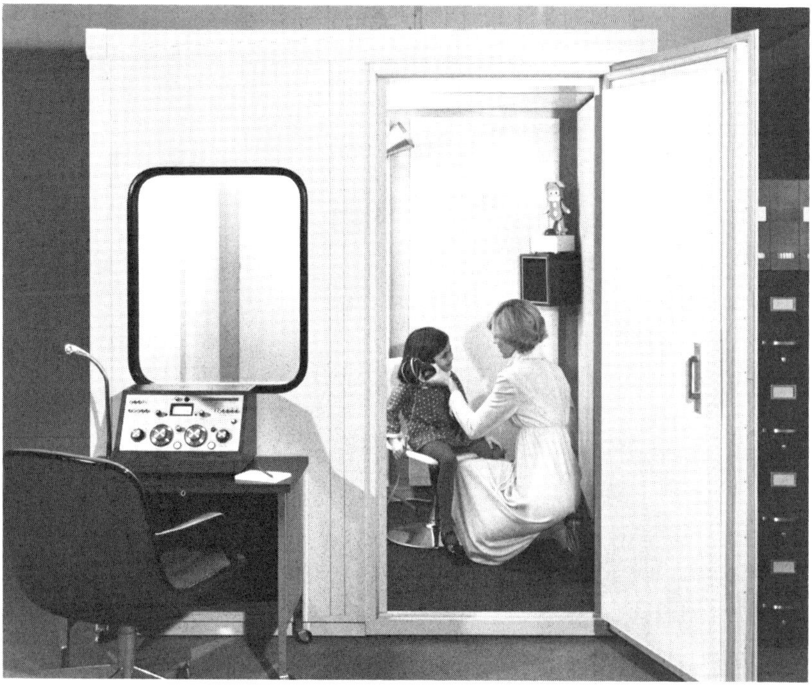

Figure 4-4. An audiometric test booth. From advertisement on the TEC II series of medical audiological rooms and suites. Cambridge, MA: Eckel Industries. Reprinted by permission.

reduced 25 dB (slight to mild loss). Then listen with sound reduced by 35, 45, 55, and 65 dB. You will be impressed with the dramatic reductions in your ability to hear the message. You will also realize that the terms for these degrees of hearing loss are misleading. The term "mild" for a 35 dB loss, for example is incorrect. A 35 dB loss is a very serious hearing loss. With a 55 dB loss, you will hardly hear the message, and with a 65 dB loss, you will not hear the message.

The effect of decreasing the frequencies ordinarily heard is also dramatic. A variable electric filter is placed between the tape recorder and the loudspeaker. The message is first heard without any filtering. Then, all frequencies above 4,000 Hz are removed. Next, all frequencies above 3000 Hz are removed. The message is understood until the filter reaches 3000 or even 2000 Hz. There is a dramatic loss of understanding when the filter setting is lowered to 1000 Hz. At 500 Hz, the

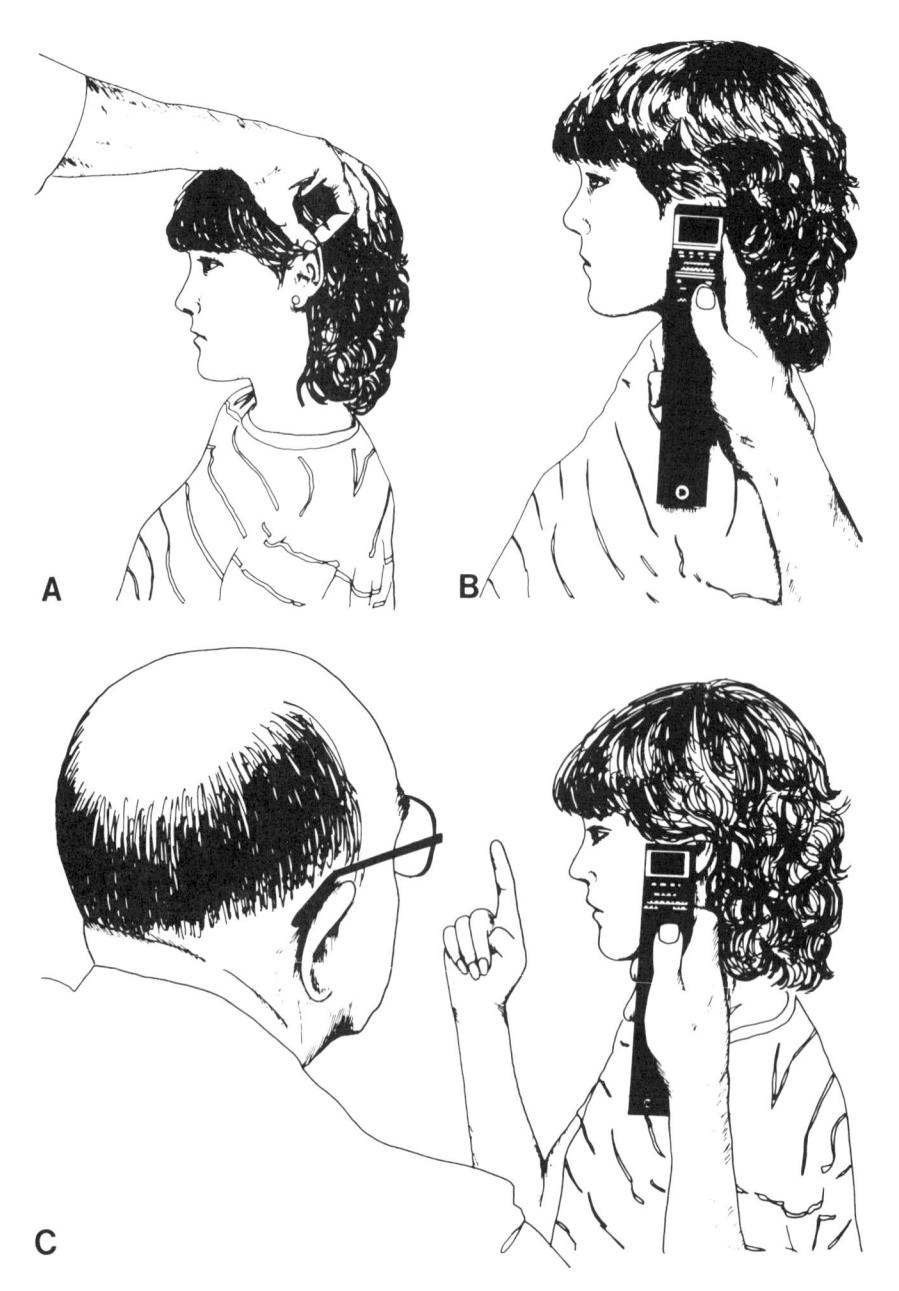

Figure 4-5. Hearing screening procedures. 1. Seat the child in a quiet room. 2. Select a speculum that will seal the ear canal. 3. Instruct the child on the method of response. 4. Turn on the audioscope. 5. Retract the auricle, as shown in A. 6. Insert the audioscope into the ear canal, as seen in B. 7. Visualize the tympanic membrane. 8. Depress the start button. 9. Observe the tone indicators and child's responses, as shown in C. 10. Screen the opposite ear. 11. Failure at any frequency necessitates rescreening. 12. A second failure indicates need for referral. Redrawn from Audioscope advertisement. Welch Allyn. Reprinted by permission.

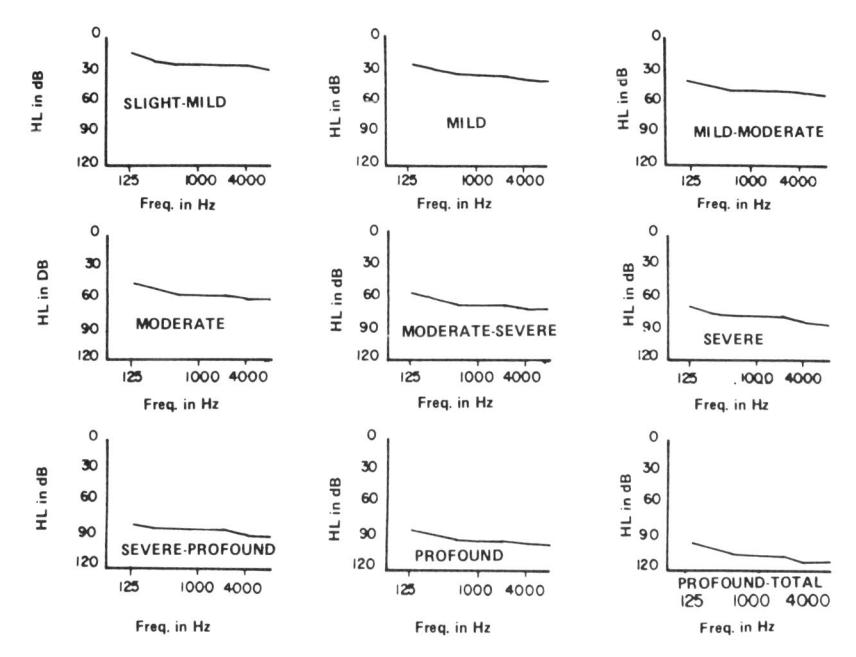

Figure 4-6. Audiograms for students with increasing hearing loss. Assume that each audiogram is a composite of audiograms for both ears. From Berg, F. (1976). *Educational audiology: Hearing and speech* (p. 40). New York: Grune & Stratton. Copyright 1976 by Grune & Stratton, Inc.

message cannot be understood, although the flow and rhythm of speech can still be recognized (Fig. 4-7).

Sensorineural hearing loss sometimes results in abrupt loss of hearing for high frequency speech sounds. Chapter 6 describes hearing aids that completely or partially restore hearing for high frequency sounds like the /s/ and /z/. It is of interest that 95 percent of speech power is located in frequencies below 1000 Hz, whereas 95 percent of speech understanding is located in frequencies above 500 Hz. Prior to listening training, it is essential that hearing impaired students have hearing aids that compensate for configuration of hearing loss. Students must be able to detect speech sounds before they can learn to recognize them.

Five-Sound Test and Earshot

A teacher can give a simple listening test to a hearing impaired student to determine how well the student hears the low, middle, and high frequencies of speech sounds. Five speech sounds representative of the frequencies and intensities of all 40 speech sounds are used. These sounds

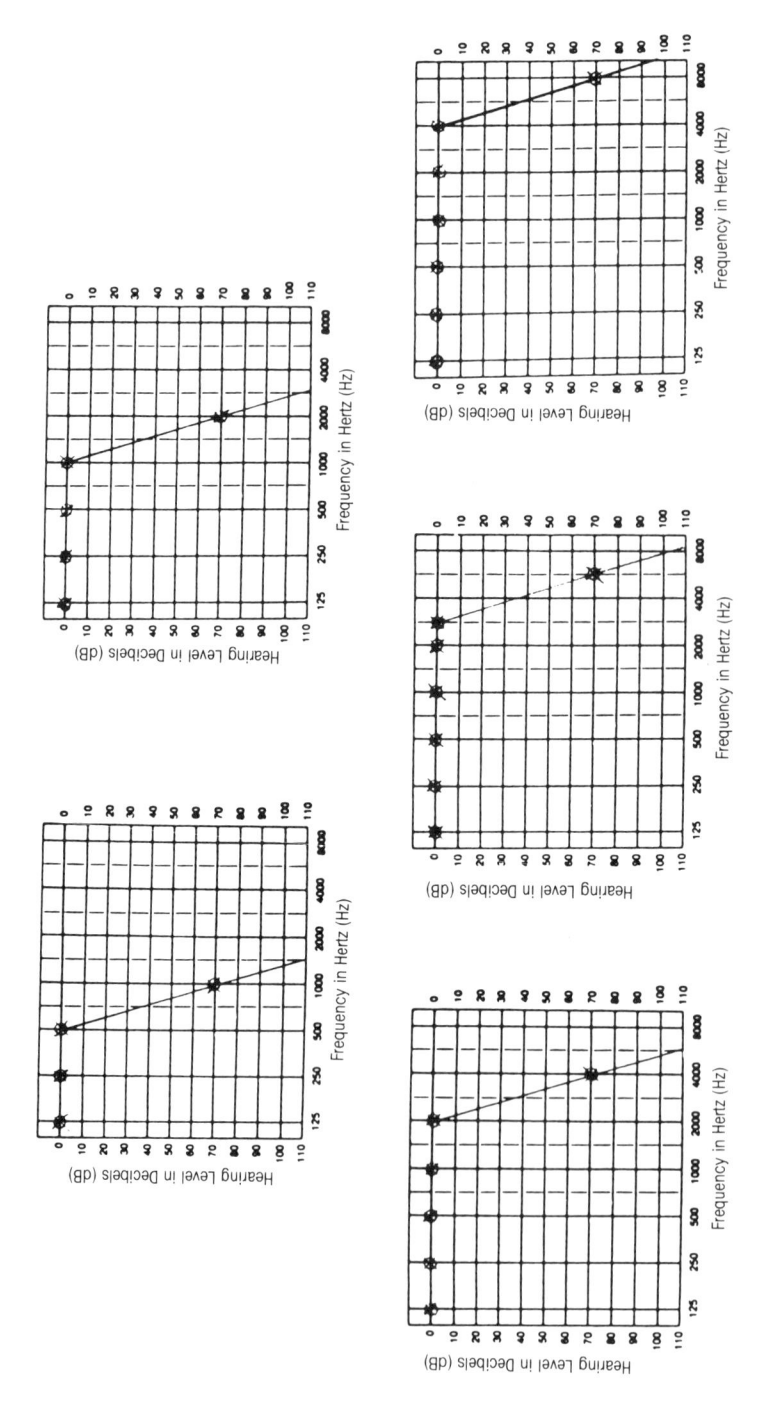

Figure 4–7. Simulated audiograms using a variable low-pass filter.

```
   1         2              3              4              5
 ╱╲       ╱╲╲          ╱╲  ╱╲          ╱╲           ╱╲
╱ u╲╲   ╱ ɑ ╲╲        ╱  ╲╱ i ╲       ╱ ʃ ╲        ╱  s ╲
 500     1000       500  2000 3000    4000          8000
```

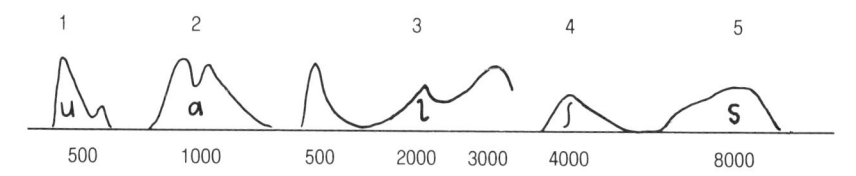

Figure 4-8. Formants of five representative speech sounds. From Ladefoged, P. (1967). *Elements of acoustic phonetics* (pp. 53, 96, 97). Chicago: University of Chicago Press. Copyright 1962 by Peter Ladefoged.

are the /u/, / ɑ /, /i/, / ʃ, and /s/. The frequency concentrations (formants) of these sounds are shown in Figure 4-8. The /u/ is concentrated at 500 Hz, the / ɑ / just below and above 1000 Hz, the /i/ at 500 Hz and just above 2000 Hz and just above 3000 Hz, the / ʃ / around 4000 Hz, and the /s/ around 8000 Hz. Hearing-impaired persons who can hear these five sounds can hear all 40 speech sounds. The test was developed by Daniel Ling.

The teacher instructs student to raise their hands if they hear the sounds. The /u/ is presented first, and then the / ɑ /, /i/, / ʃ /, and /s/ in that order. The test is given individually. The teacher and listener should be close together and in a quiet room. Optionally, the student can repeat each sound rather than indicate that it has been heard. This then becomes a speech recognition task rather than a speech detection task. Other uses of the five-sound test will be described in the following chapters.

LISTENING PROGRAM

A listening test and tasks have been developed for students with listening problems. The test includes words, sentences, and messages presented under auditory (A), visual (V), and AV conditions. On the basis of test results, tasks are selected for a student to master. The tasks also include words, sentences, and messages. The student responds to test or task items by repeating them. A speech check is given initially to determine that the trainer can understand the student's speech.

An educational audiologist, speech-language pathologist, or educator of the hearing impaired has responsibility for administering listening testing and training to students. Listening test results reveal how well students can perform initially. Table 4-1 shows listening scores for one hearing-impaired student. The results indicate that the

Table 4-1. Listening percentages of a Hard of Hearing Student under Auditory, Visual, and Auditory-Visual Conditions Using Words, Sentences, and Messages

Subtest	Auditory	Visual	Auditory-visual
Word	60	50	80
Sentence	65	60	85
Message	40	30	60

student does not listen effectively to words, sentences, or messages under either the A or V condition. Under the AV condition, the student does not perform well on messages either. AV scores are better than either A or V scores. This is expected, since the AV condition provides both auditory and lipreading cues.

The objective of listening training is to improve speech discrimination, recognition, and comprehension. Word and sentence tasks should be completed initially to build up a basic speech discrimination and recognition performance. Then, the student should be given training in comprehending messages of increasing length. Precedence is given to A training but not to the exclusion of V training. If training leads to higher A or V listening percentages, AV listening should also show improvement. Minimum desirable listening scores are 80 percent V, 90 percent A, and 95 percent AV. Discrepancies between desirable percentages and test percentages (Table 4–1) are evident.

Classroom teachers should follow the listening progress of students who have been tested and trained. A, V, and AV listening percentages should correlate with how well students can be expected to do under these same conditions in the classroom. The teacher should try to articulate speech as carefully as the specialist who is providing testing and training. If a student performs poorly under A or V conditions, the teacher should be especially aware of the need to present classroom instruction under the AV condition.

Individualized listening training provided by a specialist may take 10 to 20 hours. During and after training, the classroom teacher should also assist students in developing listening skills. The teacher can adapt regular class and individualized instruction to enhance the development of listening skills. Words, sentences, and messages should be within the language of the students.

Sentence Recognition Tasks

A teacher can make up sentence recognition tasks for class or individual practice. The sentences can be derived from regular classroom materials or common directions a teacher gives students. The vocabulary and sentence structure should be within the language capabilities of the students. The teacher or a teacher's aide can be the trainer.

Each sentence is said by a trainer and repeated by a student. If a student does not repeat back the entire sentence, the trainer should indicate the part of the sentence that is not right yet. If the sentence, for example, is *Throw me the ball* and the student repeats *Throw me a ball,* the trainer should say, *You got the first, second, and last words correct. The third word is incorrect.* The trainer should then say the sentence again, and the student repeat it again. This process should be repeated until the student says it right.

A revised ruler can serve as a visual feedback aid. The numbers 1, 2, 3, 4, 5, and so on can be spaced on the ruler. The trainer points to the numbers to indicate words correct and incorrect for each sentence missed. In the previous example, the trainer would have pointed to 1, 2, and 4 for correct and 3 for incorrect.

The trainer should go through the entire list of sentences until each sentence is repeated correctly. Then, the trainer should go back through the sentence list, following the same procedure. When a student can repeat or write down all the sentences of a list correctly on the first trial, the task is completed. Another sentence recognition task that is a little more difficult should then be presented. Increasing difficulty might simply be done by using sentence lists with more words.

Table 4–2 includes an example of a four-word sentence list and individual recording form. The number of trials needed for a student to repeat a sentence correctly may be recorded in each blank of a column. When the criterion is met, the column should include a series of ones. The total number of trials for the ten sentences may be recorded at the bottom of each column.

Table 4–2. A Four-Word Sentence Recognition Task

Stimuli	Trials per presentation time						
	1	2	3	4	5	6	7
1. Throw me the ball.	___	___	___	___	___	___	___
2. Jump off the bench.	___	___	___	___	___	___	___
3. Hand it to him.	___	___	___	___	___	___	___
4. Sing us a song.	___	___	___	___	___	___	___
5. I saw him come.	___	___	___	___	___	___	___
6. A chimp is funny.	___	___	___	___	___	___	___
7. Bill needs a shot.	___	___	___	___	___	___	___
8. Turn on the light.	___	___	___	___	___	___	___
9. His socks are red.	___	___	___	___	___	___	___
10. Joan loves bright colors.	___	___	___	___	___	___	___
Totals	___	___	___	___	___	___	___

Message Tasks

A teacher can also adapt regular instructional materials into message tasks. An example of a message task appears here. The teacher or an aide says the entire message. A student of class answers questions afterwards to test message comprehension. Student responses can be spoken or written. The message can be repeated until all questions are answered correctly.

Message: A hippopotamus may weigh 5000 pounds. It can walk on the bottom of a river.

Questions: 1. What kind of animal? _____ (hippopotamus)
2. It may weigh? _____ (5000 pounds)
3. It can do what? _____ (walk)
4. Where does it walk? _____ (in a river)
5. Where in a river? _____ (on the bottom)

Instructional material can be divided into a series of as many as 50 messages. The division points should be set so that short messages occur first and then increasingly longer messages. The number of concepts per message might increase from 5 to as many as 40.

Self-Instruction

To reach full capacity in listening, the student needs extensive practice. Normally this practice is provided through incidental daily learning experiences provided by the environment with no special teaching or learning effort. With hearing impaired students, a formal listening curriculum is needed. Self-instruction with a tape recorder can be included after listening tasks have been introduced through "live" instruction.

A student using FM equipment can tape record a teacher's lesson. This tape recording will be of high quality because the FM equipment bypasses room noise. The student can play back the recording and listen to the lesson as many times as desirable. This listening activity will provide useful auditory training. The student can take notes, and the teacher or aide checks them to determine how well the lesson has been understood.

Much of the special listening instruction of specialists can also be self-instructional. This includes basic prosodic discrimination tasks, more difficult word recognition tasks, and very difficult phonetic discrimination tasks.

Computer assisted instruction is also becoming available to train specialists and teachers to give listening tests and tasks. One computer program, for example, provides training recommendations based on test results. It initially computes percentages of correct responses on each subtest and displays a summary of subtest percentage scores.

Videotape and videodisc listening materials will also become available. The student will be able to switch from visual to auditory to auditory-visual training as desirable. The student will also be able to quickly access any listening task by checking an index and pushing a number.

SUMMARY

Effective listening is basic to school learning. Each child with any degree of hearing loss is at listening risk. Many children with normal hearing also have listening problems. Hearing impaired children do not listen effectively because they cannot detect or recognize many of the speech sounds. The audiogram and the five-sound test are useful predictors of speech detection ability. A listening test provides data on speech recognition ability. Hearing screening is effective for identifying children with possible hearing loss. Various types of listening tasks can be given by specialists and teachers or their aides, through "live"—or self-instruction. Early and continuing listening instruction enhances classroom learning. Auditory and visual (lipreading) training should be given as needed.

FURTHER READINGS

Erik Wedenberg's monograph article "Auditory Training of Severely Hard of Hearing Pre-School Children" (*Acta Otolaryngologica,* Supplementum 110, Stockholm, 1954) is the classic reference on developmental listening training. Doreen Pollack's *Educational Audiology for the Infant and Preschooler* (Charles C. Thomas, Springfield, IL, 1985) is an equally important reference on developmental listening training. Thomas Clark and Susan Watkin's *Programming for Hearing Impaired Infants through Amplification and Home Intervention* (Utah State University, Logan, UT, 1985) provides practical developmental listening tasks. The *Auditory Instructional Planning System* of Los Angeles County (Forewarks, North Hollywood, CA) includes a standardized Test of Auditory Comprehension (TAC) and auditory training curriculum for hearing-impaired children 4 to 12 years old with losses greater than 55 dB. An auditory, visual, and auditory-visual listening test and word, sentence, and message tasks, called *Listening*

Refinement Program (Smithfield, UT, 1986) has been developed by Frederick Berg and Dee Child. Frederick Berg's book *Educational Audiology: Hearing and Speech Management* (Grune & Stratton, New York, 1976) summarizes previous listening training programs for children and adults.

APPENDIX

Sound Intensity

Each separate sound has an intensity that is expressed in decibels (dB) based on powers of 10. The difference in intensity between the faintest sound that can be normally heard (0 dB) and the loudest sound that can be normally tolerated (120 dB) is 10 × 10 × 10 × 10 × 10 × 10 × 10 × 10 × 10 × 10 × 10 × 10 to 1, or 1 trillion to one. A 10 db increase is 10 times the intensity of the original value: 20 dB 100 times, 30 dB 1000 times, etc. A hearing loss decreases the intensity range of sounds that can be heard from 1 trillion to 1 to less, depending on degree of loss. Table 4–3 clarifies the decibel by relating it to familiar sound intensity conditions. A person with a 60 dB hearing loss and without a hearing aid, for example, barely hears quiet conversation at 1 meter. That person would not hear soft whisper background noise in a quiet room, but would hear loud classroom noise and shouts.

Sound intensity is a physical phenomenon that can be measured with a sound level meter. As sound intensity changes, people perceive the change as a change in loudness. People hear sounds in loudness units called sones. (Ladefoged, 1967; Stevens and Davis, 1938).

Table 4–3. Decibels, Powers of 10 Ratios, and Faint to Loud Conditions

dB	Ratio	Condition
0	1:1	Normal hearing threshold at ear
20	100:1	Soft whisper at 1 meter
40	10,000:1	Background noise in quiet room
60	1,000,000:1	Quiet conversation at 1 meter
80	100,000,000:1	Very noisy classroom
100	10,000,000,000:1	Shout at 1 meter
120	1,000,000,000,000:1	Shout next to ear

Frequency of Sound

Sound is vibration that can be heard. The rate or frequency of vibration that can be normally heard by a child varies from 16 cycles per second (cps) to 16,000 cps. The unit of frequency is the hertz (Hz), the same as cps. Whereas spaces along the intensity scale are expressed in decibels, based on powers of 10, spaces along the frequency scale are expressed in Hz, based on powers of 2, a doubling relationship. The doubling ratio is shown as equal intervals along the frequency scale of Table 4-4. A person with a sensorineural hearing loss without a hearing aid typically does not hear very high frequencies and often does not hear all the high frequencies.

People perceive frequency as pitch. The pitch of middle C on the piano keyboard is a result of a fundamental frequency of vibration of 256 Hz. One octave above middle C is 512 Hz; one octave below, 128 Hz. The piano keyboard extends somewhat more than seven octaves. The lowest note is between 16 and 32 Hz. The highest note is just above 4096 Hz. Whereas frequency is expressed in Hz units, pitch is expressed in mel units.

Air and Bone Conduction Testing

Ordinarily, sound from an audiometer is delivered to the ear of a person through an earphone. The sound is conducted through the entire ear, including the ear canal, middle ear, and inner ear, to the brain stems and cortices. This test procedure provides air conduction detection thresholds. Hearing loss will be evident if it exists. Air conduction testing, however, does not indicate the location of any pathologic condition.

Many audiometers, however, make provision for sound to be delivered through a vibrator placed against the bone of the head. Sound bypasses the outer and middle ears and is delivered directly to the cochlea, where it moves on to the brain stems and cortices. This test procedure provides bone conduction detection thresholds. If the same degree of hearing loss is still evident, the test indicates that the pathology is in the cochlea, the brain stem, or one or both cortices. If hearing loss is evident but substantially less, the hearing loss is mixed.

Table 4-4. Frequency Scale for Sounds in Hz

16	32	64	128	256	512	1024	2048	4096	8192	16,384
Low					Middle		High			Very High

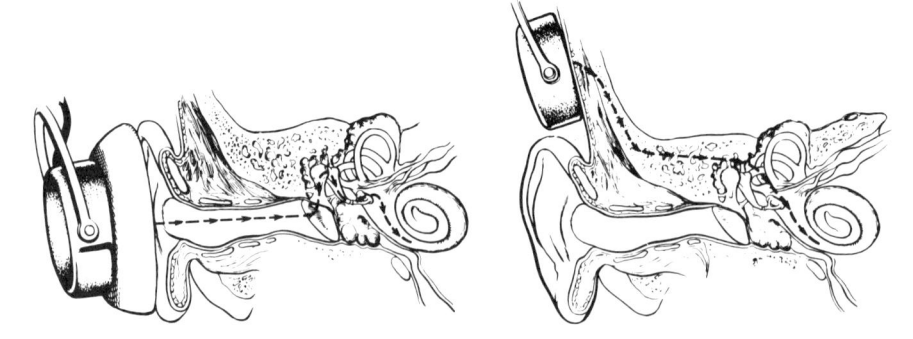

Figure 4-9. Air conduction testing (left) and bone conduction testing (right). From Zenith Hearing Aid Sales Corporation. (1965). Zenith Training Course, Unit 7, Conductive and Sensorineural Hearing Impairments (p. 3), Chicago. Copyright 1965 by Zenith Hearing Aid Sales Corporation. Reprinted by permission.

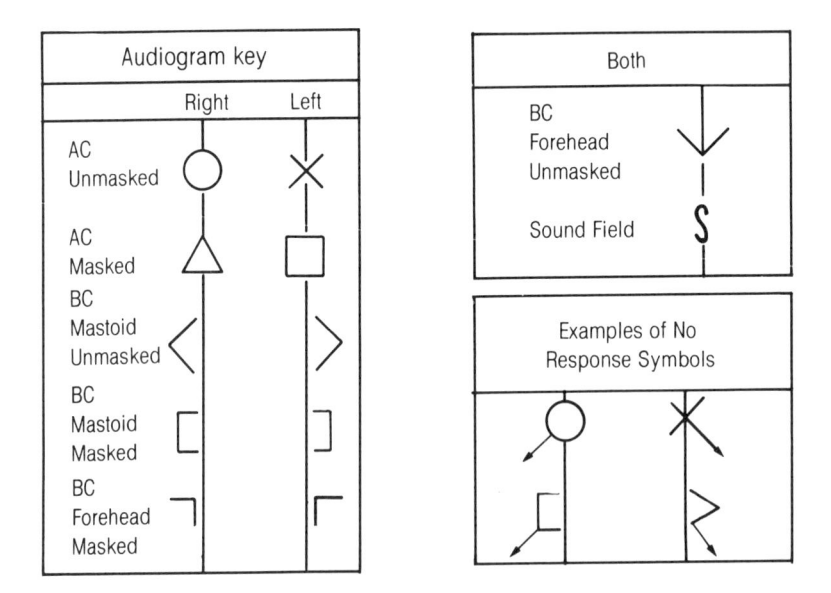

Figure 4-10. Audiogram symbols used to explain test conditions or responses. From Committee on Audiometric Evaluation. (1974). Guidelines for audiometric symbols. *ASHA, 17,* 260-264. Copyright 1974 by the American Speech-Language-Hearing Association. Reprinted by permission.

Figure 4-11. See page 86 for legend.

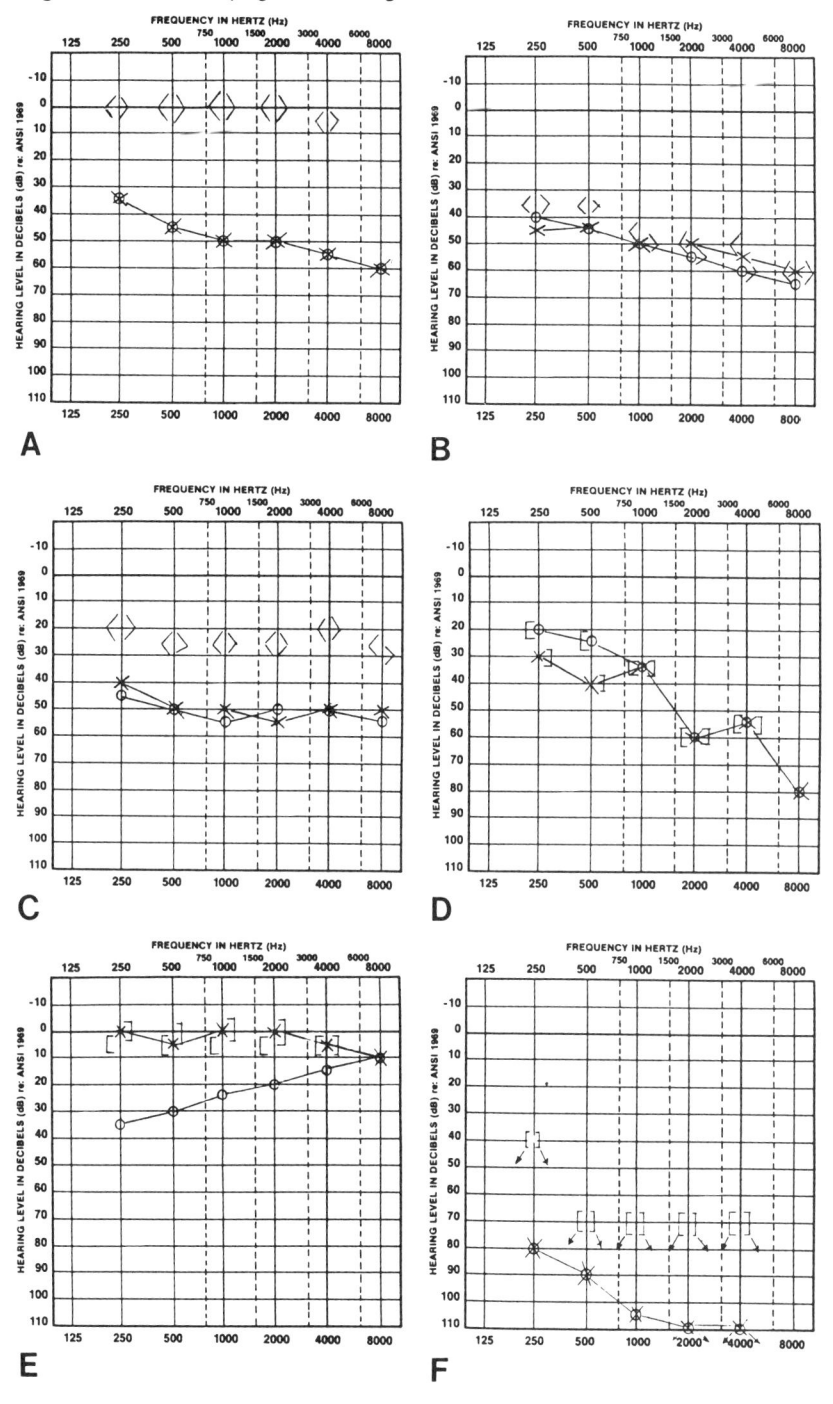

86 Facilitating Classroom Listening

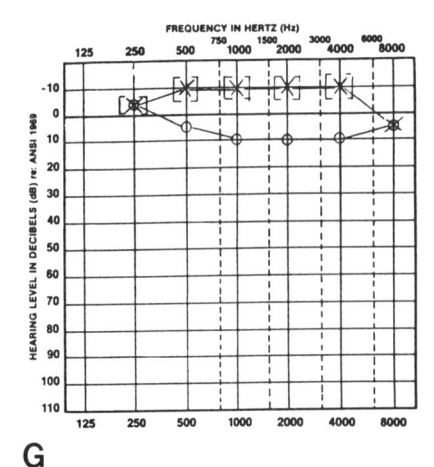

Figure 4-11. Audiograms for different hearing impairments. (a) Conductive bilateral loss. (b) Sensorineural bilateral loss. (c) Mixed bilateral loss. (d) High tone sensorineural loss. (e) Low tone conductive unilateral (right) loss. (f) Near-total sensorineural bilateral loss. (g) Slight conductive unilateral (right) loss.

Air conduction testing through an earphone is done first, and if a loss occurs, bone conduction testing through a vibrator is then done. Figure 4–9 illustrates air and bone conducted sound input to an ear. Other hearing tests are performed to assist in determining whether the condition is cochlear, in the brain stem, or in cortices.

Sometimes during air conduction testing and often during bone conduction testing, a masking sound is purposely introduced into the nontest ear. When a masking sound is used, the nontest ear will be kept from detecting the tone introduced into the test ear. In this way, only the ear being tested will contribute to the determination of detection thresholds. Masking is especially used in bone conduction testing because a sound introduced by a bone vibrator will reach the cochleas of both ears equally well. This is because there is no loss of energy from one side of the head to the other side with bone conducted sound. In fact, the vibrator may be placed on the mastoid bone behind one ear and the sound sensed in the opposite cochlea at a lower detection level, if the opposite cochlea is less impaired.

Different symbols are used to indicate unmasked and masked air and bone conduction thresholds. Figure 4–10 shows the symbols recommended by ASHA (1974). A red color keys a right ear response. A blue color indicates a left ear response. The most commonly used symbols are circles for the right ear and crosses for the left ear. Lines are drawn to connect symbols to produce audiograms. The symbols for bone conduction thresholds are drawn to the left or right of intersection points. A symbol to the left on the audiogram form indicates a right ear response, with the understanding that the listener is facing the tester. A symbol to the right, correspondingly, indicates a left ear response (Hodgson, 1980).

Interpreting Audiograms

Air and bone conduction audiograms provide detection and information about the site of pathologic conditions for medical, amplification, and listening intervention. Seven sample audiograms are shown here (Fig. 4–11). The bone conduction detection thresholds for the sixth audiogram indicate that the upper intensity limits of the audiometer for bone conducted sound had been reached.

Chapter 5

Room Acoustics

CASE STUDY

AJ is a 17 year old senior high school student who has just transferred schools. She has a bilateral hearing loss. She says she is having more difficulty understanding than she did in her previous school. In the other school the kids were quieter and the rooms were sound treated. There was also more discipline and the kids could concentrate better. AJ is a good student and wants to get a university scholarship. She is particularly interested in science.

AJ has worn a hearing aid for most of her life. She says her hearing aid worked originally all right but now picks up a lot of noise at school. She has found it does not help to turn up the volume control of the aid any further. The hearing aid just picks up that much more noise. Her aid is fairly new and has a special noise suppressor. The suppressor helps at home but not at the new school.

AJ's father is an acoustical engineer. He specializes in reducing noise and reverberation. He has shown AJ how to use a sound level meter and has told her to take it to school and make measurements. AJ has recorded the following decibel levels in her classrooom: unoccupied 50, occupied with students 60 to 80, fan without students 70, overhead projector without students 65, teacher's voice at 1 meter 65, teacher's voice at 4 meters 59 dB. Other decibel levels in the school are as follows: hallway 75, auditorium 80, cafeteria 85, gymnasium 90, wood shop 95, body and fender shop 100 dB.

Alarmed at the results, AJ's father makes an appointment to visit the school. Upon arriving he notes that the school building is located on a heavily traveled street. A lot of students ride motorcycles, and some have cars with noisy mufflers. A number of classroom windows to the outside are open. Some of the outside doors of the school have been left open.

AJ's father also notices that the students are permitted to make a lot of noise in the halls. Students are not quiet in the classrooms, either. The principal believes in a "democratic" school. Sometimes the students are really boisterous.

Another thing he finds is that the classrooms in the school have very little acoustical treatment. There is acoustical tile but no rugs or drapes. The hallways, auditorium, cafeteria, and gymnasium are all hard surfaced. No sound barriers exist in the shops or other rooms where heavy equipment and tools are used.

Maintenance repairs are also needed. Ventilating ductwork and plumbing pipes vibrate. Room fans need to be oiled. Projectors need servicing.

AJ's father talks to the principal about the noise and reverberation problems he has noticed and the consequent listening and hearing aid difficulties AJ is having in school. The principal listens carefully. He expresses concern with the acoustical problems. He tells AJ's father that the school has been operating on a very restricted budget for the last 5 years because of continuous cutbacks in state school funds. He asks AJ to serve on a committee to study the problem further and make recommendations to the school board. The principal cannot promise miracles, but he believes improvements can be made. AJ's father accepts the committee position and agrees to offer his equipment and services without charge for the study.

During the next month the committee is set up. Members of the committee include the principal (chairman), AJ's father, the head custodian, two teachers, the student body president, and the district educational audiologist. Sound measurement equipment is used to take noise and reverberation measurements in various school locations. During the next 3 months a report is written with recommendations for change. A series of administrative, teacher, school board, and parent meetings are held to discuss the findings and recommendations. Later that year, AJ reports she is doing well and can understand better in school.

BASICS OF ACOUSTICS

Importance and Problem

Room acoustics often affect listening in a negative way. Room noise, room reverberation, and talker-listener distance are factors of this problem. These variables affect listening effectiveness of normal hearing students and especially hard of hearing students. Currently, classroom acoustics are a widespread problem in regular and special schools of this country. The objective of this chapter is to describe classroom acoustics and what can be done to alleviate their adverse effects. Basic definitions and processes are explained first, then the impact of room acoustics upon listening, next measurement procedures, and last alleviation considerations.

Definitions and Processes

Sound is propagated vibration that can be heard. Each cycle of vibration of a sound source causes like vibrations of air molecules adjacent to the source. These in turn cause a corresponding vibration in the next layer of air molecules. An expanding sphere of countless billions of air molecules is set into vibration in a chain reaction. Figure 5-1 shows how compressed and spread molecules cause positive (upward) and negative (downward) parts of each successive wave form.

Simultaneously, sound waves propagate outward in all directions with a speed of 1129 feet per second in air. Sound waves, like water waves, are spread over an increasingly expanding area. A new wave is propagated with each successive cycle of vibration of the sound source. Correspondingly, sound intensity decreases in decibels as sound waves travel further from their source, like the receding crests of water waves seen in Figure 5-1.

When propagated sound meets a partition (wall, ceiling, or floor) or room barrier, it is affected in several ways. Part of the sound is absorbed, part is reflected, part passes through (transmitted), and, with a barrier, part is diffracted. The softer the partition or barrier surface, the more sound will be absorbed. The harder the surface, the more sound will be reflected. The less dense the partition or barrier, the more sound will be transmitted through it. The further away and lower the barrier, the more sound will be diffracted or bent around it. Figure 5-2 diagrams these effects and shows unobstructed direct sound propagation.

When a room has hard surfaces, propagated sound from a source reflects repeatedly from the walls, ceiling, and floor. Repeated reflection causes prolongation of sound, which is called reverberation. In a room, direct sound and reflected or reverberated sound reach a listener. In detail, there is a direct sound, early reflections, and closed, packed, later reflections (Fig. 5-3).

Reverberant sound interferes with listening to direct sound. The longer it takes for reverberation to cease, the more the listening interference. If the sound source is speech, the direct speech sound is smeared or masked by the reverberant speech sound. This reverberant effect can be understood by the first speech sound of a word smearing the second

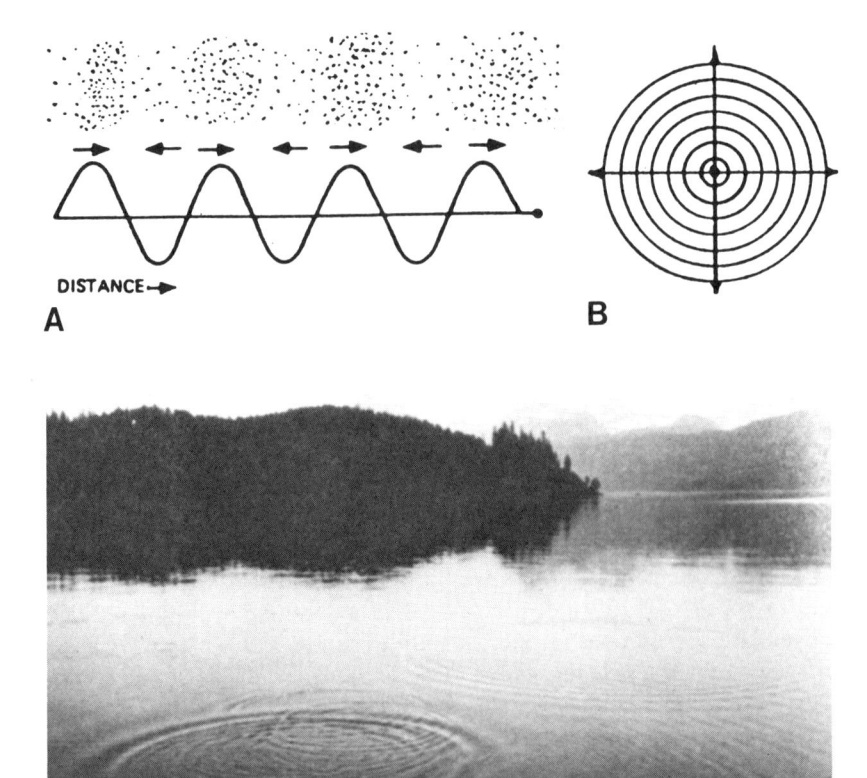

Figure 5-1. (A) Schematization of molecules and wave forms. From Goldstein, J. (1978). Fundamental concepts in sound measurement. In D. Lipscomb (Ed.), *Noise and audiology,* Baltimore: University Park Press. Copyright 1978 by University Park Press. Reprinted by permission. (B) An expanding wave front from a sound source. (C) Water waves. From Amend, J. (1983). *Physics.* Englewood Cliffs, NJ: Prentice-Hall. Copyright 1983 by Prentice-Hall, Inc. Reprinted by permission.

speech sound of that word. The second speech sound in turn smears the third speech sound, and so on. The longer the reverberation, the more widespread the smearing effect. One speech sound may smear not only the following speech sound of a word but the two or three speech sounds that follow. Vowel sounds particularly smear consonant sounds because (1) vowels are more intense and (2) the higher frequencies that characterize many consonants are often absorbed more effectively by room surfaces.

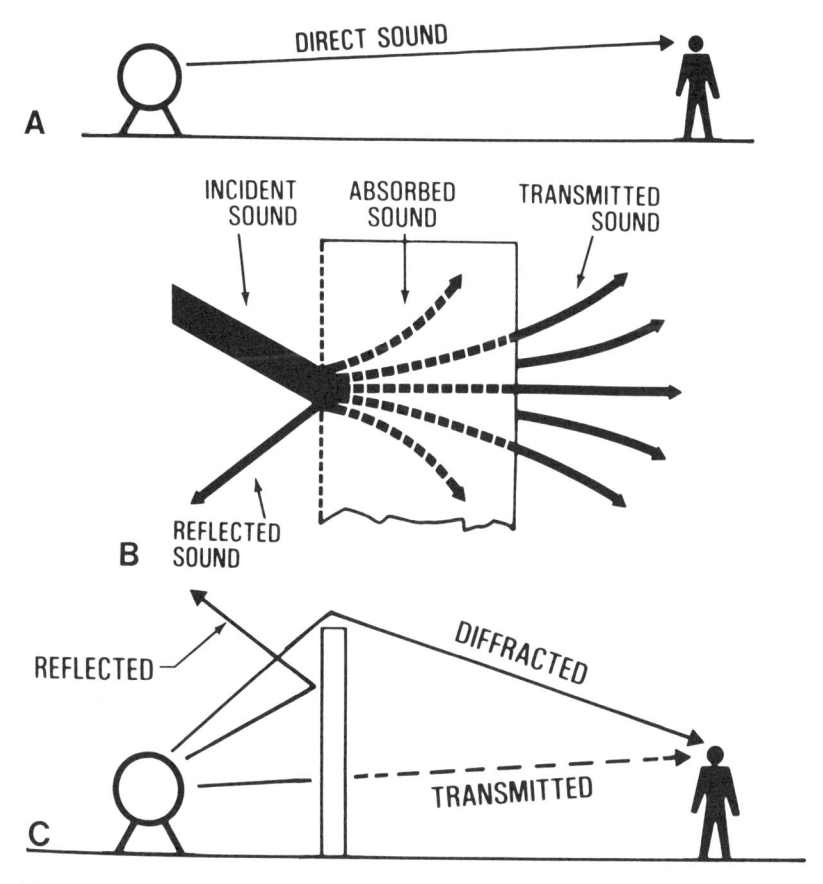

Figure 5-2. (A) Direct propagation of sound between a sound source and a listener. (B) The breaking of a sound path by a partition. (C) The effect of placing a barrier between the source and the listener. (From Hirshorn, M. (1982). *IAC noise control handbook* (pp. C-6, C-5, C-7). Bronx, NY: Industrial Acoustics Company. Copyright 1982 by Industrial Acoustics Company. Reprinted by permission.)

Reverberation can be measured by the time it takes a sound to stop reflecting. Reverberation time (RT) is the time in seconds required for a sound that is produced to reduce 60 dB in intensity once that sound is no longer being generated. A hard room has a long RT, whereas a soft (absorbent) room has a short RT.

The RT of a room alters the effect of the speaker-listener distance upon sound intensity. In a room with a RT of 0, sound intensity decreases 6 dB with every doubling of distance. If the sound intensity is 65 dB at 1 meter from the sound source (speaker), it is 59 dB at 2 meters, 53 dB at 4 meters, and 47 dB at 8 meters. As the RT of a room

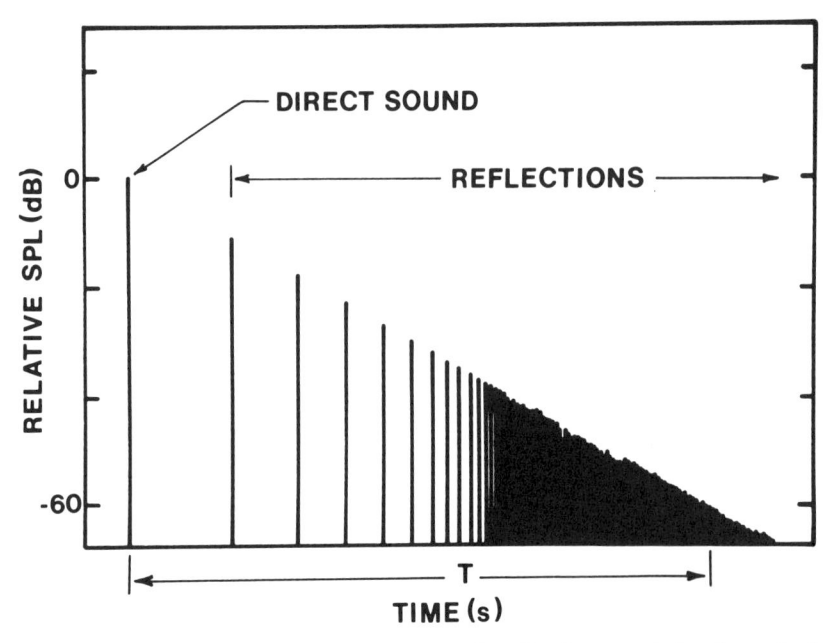

Figure 5-3. Schematic of direct sound, early reflections, and closely packed reverberant sound. (From Nabelek, A., and Nabalek, F. (1985). Room acoustics and speech perception (p. 835). In J. Katz (Ed.) *Handbook of clinical audiology*. Baltimore: Williams & Wilkins. Copyright 1985 by Williams & Wilkins. Reprinted by permission.)

increased from 0 to more than 1 second, the decrease of sound intensity with increase of speaker-listener distance is less and less. Figure 5–4 shows the relationship between decibel level and distance from source in meters for increasing RTs. The diagonal line shows the 6 dB decrease per doubling of distance for direct sound. The curve for 10 k (10,000 sabins of absorption or a very short RT) also shows a considerable decibel decrease for each doubling of distance. The top or 50 sabins curve (a very long RT) shows only a slight decibel decrease for each doubling of speaker-listener distance.

It might seem from the preceding description that it is desirable to have a high RT, but this is not so. It is true that sound can be detected more easily at longer distances with a high RT, but that sound will also be smeared more. A better option is to have a low RT with little or no smearing and to amplify the sound with a hearing aid or public address system, or even better, transmit it to listeners with FM equipment that will be described in Chapter 7.

The final room acoustic problem is noise. Acoustical noise is any unwanted sound. The school environment is filled with various noises

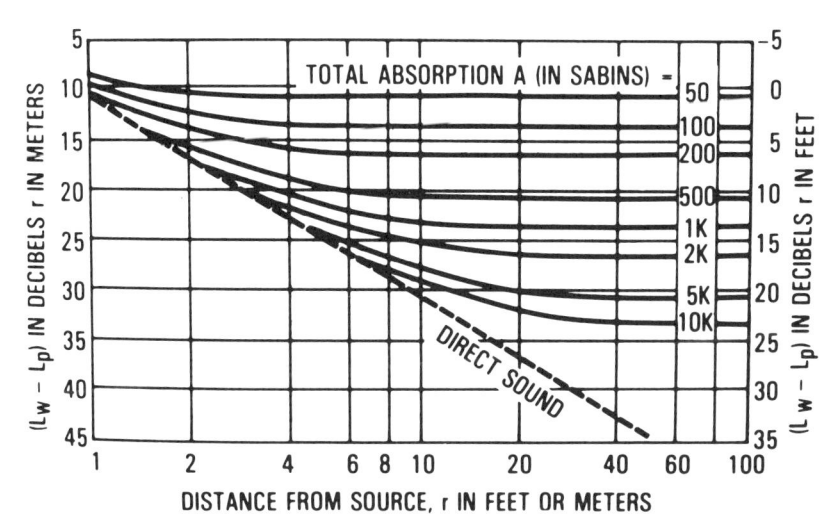

Figure 5-4. Sound intensity decrease in decibels with increasing distance from sound source under different reverberant conditions. (From Waterhouse, R., and Harris, C. (1979). Sound in enclosed spaces (p. 4-9). In C. Harris (Ed.) *Handbook of noise control.* New York: McGraw-Hill. Copyright 1979 by McGraw-Hill Book Company, Inc. Reprinted by permission.)

from myriad sources. Even at night, when a classroom is unoccupied and supposedly quiet, background noise is present. This noise may be referred to as the noise floor. Decibel levels within the noise floor are greatest for the lower frequencies and become progressively less at higher and higher frequencies. During the day, and particularly when the space is occupied, the noise floor increases in overall intensity, and in high-frequency composition because of the inclusion of human voices, particularly children's voices.

The sound we desire to hear is not a part of the noise floor. It is referred to as the signal. The teacher's voice, for example is called the speech signal. The speech signal includes all of the speech sounds of words and sentences used by the teacher to instruct students. The individual decibel levels within the speech signal also progressively become less and less from the low frequencies to the high frequencies, although noise extends lower in frequency than the speech signal does. Figure 5–5 shows the dB levels and frequencies of the noise floor of a classroom and the speech spectra (signal) of adult male and female speakers.

The noise and signal each have an overall decibel value. The difference between the signal in decibels and the noise in decibels is called the signal-to-noise (S/N) ratio. The S/N ratio is also referred to as the message-to-competition ratio. To a teacher trying to get a message across

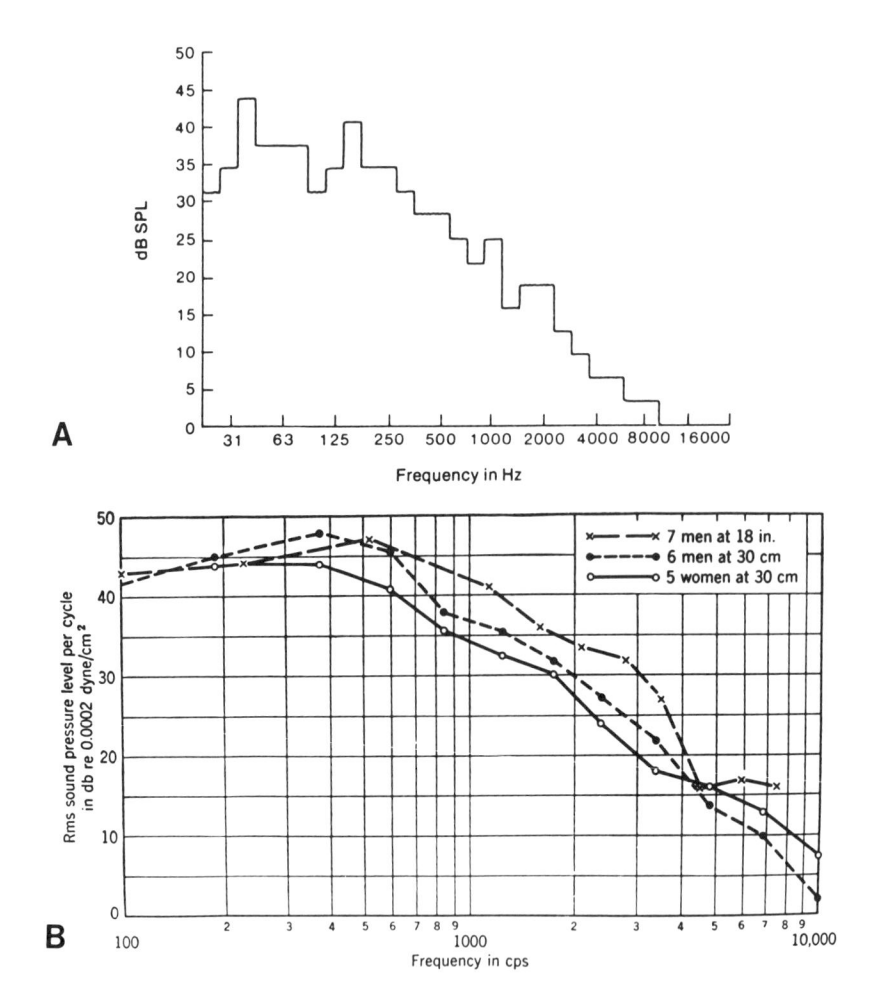

Figure 5-5. (A) The noise floor of an unoccupied classroom. (From Berg, F., et al. (1983). *Listening in classrooms, hard of hearing* (p. 11). Logan: Utah State University. Reprinted by permission.) (B) The speech spectra of adult males and females at 10 to 30" from the speech source. (From Licklider, J., and Miller, G. (1951). The perception of speech (p. 1042). In S. Stevens (Ed.) *Handbook of experimental psychology.* New York: John Wiley & Sons. Copyright 1951 by John Wiley & Sons, Inc. Reprinted by permission.)

to a class, the competition may be traffic noise or children talking or otherwise disturbing the classroom. A S/N ratio of 0 dB means that both the signal and the noise have the same intensity. A S/N ratio of +10 dB means the signal is 10 dB more intense than the noise. A S/N ratio of −10 dB means that the noise is 10 dB more intense than the signal. When a person puts on a hearing aid, both the signal level and the noise level are heard more intensely. The S/N ratio may stay where it was without sound amplification. If the S/N was undesirable without an aid, it is still undesirable with the aid.

CLASSROOM LISTENING DATA

Differences in classroom noise and RT influence the degree to which students can understand a teacher. The typical school classroom has an occupied noise level of 60 dBA or more and a RT of more than 0.4 seconds, both of which are undesirable, particularly for students with hearing loss. The effects are illustrated in Table 5–1, which presents speech recognition scores of school age children under several noise and reverberation conditions. Listening scores are compared at 0.4 and 1.2 second RTs and with S/N ratios of 0, +6, and +12 dB. The students with normal hearing had mean speech recognition scores of 95 percent, and the hard of hearing students had mean scores of 83 percent, when tested in an audiometric test booth with negligible noise and reverberation.

The 0.4 and 1.2 second RTs simulate classrooms with considerable and minimal acoustical treatment, respectively. The +12 dB S/N ratio has been considered minimally acceptable for a hard of hearing student

Table 5-1. Average Speech Recognition Scores of 12 Normal Hearing and 12 Hard of Hearing Students under RTs and S/N Ratios Simulating Various Classroom Conditions

RTs (in seconds)	S/N ratios (in dB)	Percentage of words repeated Normal	H-of-H
0.4	+12	83	60
	+6	71	52
	0	48	28
1.2	+12	70	41
	+6	54	27
	0	30	11

From Finitzo-Hieber, T. (1981). Classroom acoustics. In R. Roesner and M. Downs (Eds.). *Auditory disorders in school children.* New York: Thieme-Stratton. Copyright 1981 by Thieme-Stratton.

in a classroom (Gengel, 1971). The +6 and 0 dB S/N ratios are fairly typical of school classrooms. The scores of Table 5-1 reveal that even students with normal hearing cannot listen optimally in a typically noisy school classroom, even when the room has considerable acoustical treatment.

The "hard of hearing" data in Table 5-1 are for students with bilateral hearing loss. It is likely that the listening scores of students with unilateral hearing loss would fall somewhere between the scores of normal hearing students and the scores of students with unilateral hearing loss. In a recent laboratory study, Bess (1982) found that students with bilateral hearing loss experience learning difficulties in classrooms, even when given preferential seating (teacher facing normal ear of student).

Perusal of the data in Table 5-1 indicates that both noise and reverberation deleteriously affect listening scores, and that the combination of both is especially detrimental. The listening scores were obtained at a 12 foot distance, simulating class instruction. Only in the immediate vicinity of the teacher can students listen only to direct sound. At a 12 foot distance, students hear both direct and reverberant sound.

Optimal RTs for hard of hearing students are lower than for normal hearing students. Hard of hearing students might listen more effectively if RT is reduced to 0, provided the sound signal is amplified so they can hear it well. Students with normal hearing might listen optimally if RT is reduced to 0.1 to 0.2 seconds, provided they can hear the signal well.

Optimal S/N levels are 30+ dB for hard of hearing students and 20+ dB for students with normal hearing. The speech signal will vary from 65 dBA at 1 meter to decreasing levels at greater teacher-student distances, depending on RT. Ideally, classrooms should be quiet. The dBA noise level during academic instruction should be 35 dBA or less. Perhaps a more practical criterion for minimum noise level is 50 dBA for an occupied classroom. In a recent study of fairly modern classrooms used by elementary and junior high students, unoccupied noise levels of 41 dBA and occupied noise levels of 56 dBA were found.

MEASUREMENT AND CALCULATION

Instruments are available for measurement of signal and noise in decibels and RT in seconds. A complete battery-operated system for programming, taking and printing sound measurements is shown in Figure 5-6. This fully portable system can automatically measure (1) intensity levels from −10 to 140 dB at various frequencies from 1 to 20,000 Hz and (2) RTs at various frequencies.

Room Acoustics 99

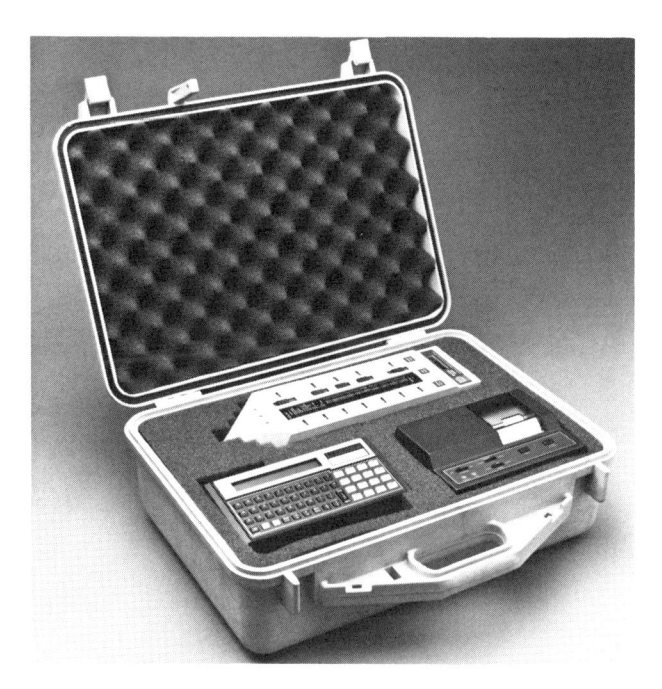

Figure 5-6. Larson-Davis Model 800B sound level meter in carrying case with computer printer, and mass memory unit. (From Larson-Davis advertisement. Pleasant Grove, UT: Larson-Davis Laboratories. Reprinted by permission.)

A time history of sound intensity in decibels can be obtained with a docimeter. Figure 5-7 shows a docimeter with printer that scores and graphs time-sampled measures of sound intensity in ½ dB steps from 35 to 145 dBA. Up to 2 weeks of data may be stored in the meter before printing.

A docimeter may be worn by a mobile person or placed in a stationary location. Docimeter measures on a 13 year old boy during a school day are shown in Figure 5-8. The docimeter was worn continually by the boy from the time he got up one morning to later that evening. Measurements were taken automatically every 3 minutes. The horizontal bars are hourly averages. This docimeter was not designed to read below 60 dBA. The sound intensity levels exceeded 60 dBA the great majority of the time and 90 dBA at times. The readings were from signals and noises produced by the boy and other persons and by noise sources in and out of school. Note particularly the intense dBA levels encountered by the boy on the school bus or while he was eating lunch. In a rowdy science class, the levels exceeded 80 dBA.

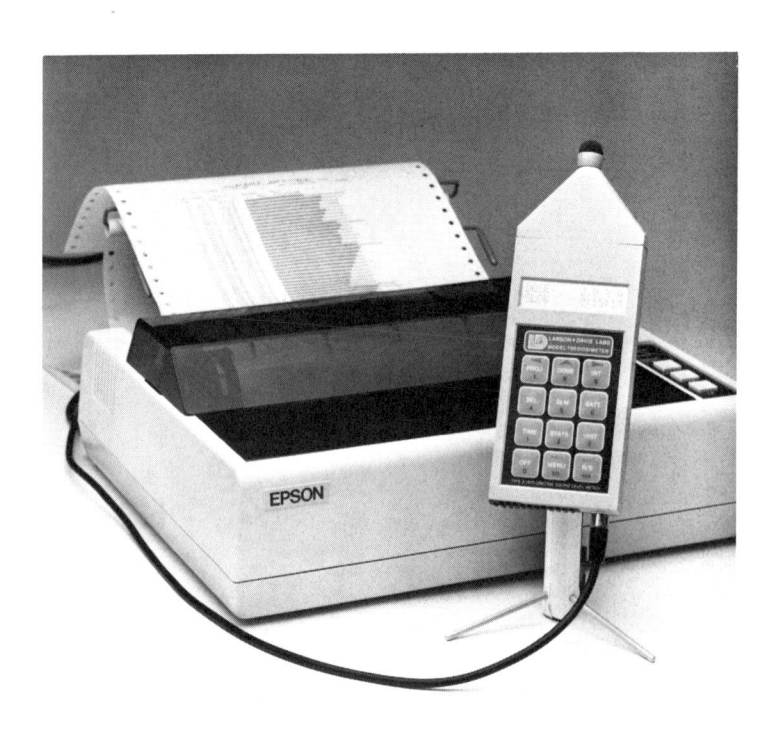

Figure 5-7. Larson-Davis Model 700 docimeter/sound level meter and Epson printer. (From Larson-Davis advertisement. Pleasant Grove, UT: Larson-Davis Laboratories. Reprinted by permission.)

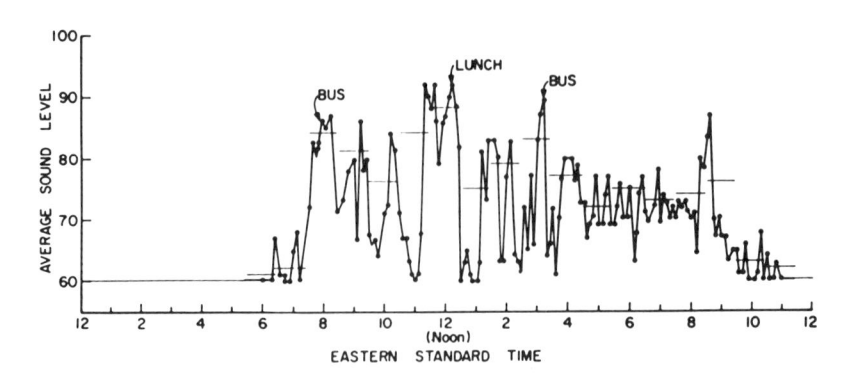

Figure 5-8. Docimeter measures on a 13 year old boy during a school day. (From *Why is the noise dose of humans important?* Unpublished presentation. Dayton, OH: Wright-Patterson Air Force Base, Aerospace Medical Research Laboratory, 1979. Reprinted by permission.)

Sound intensity can be measured with A, B, or C scales. The A scale is used when considering the impact of sound intensity upon a person. This is because the dBA response of the meter compensates for less sensitive human hearing at lower frequencies. On the A scale the meter shuts out frequencies of the noise floor below the frequencies used for detecting speech sounds. On the B scale the meter shuts out less low frequency energy. On the C scale the meter lets in low frequency sounds as well as middle and high frequency sounds (Fig. 5–9).

The precision sound level meter and the docimeter are instruments used by engineers and audiologists. A simpler meter, of very low cost, can be used by a teacher to measure overall sound intensities from 50 to 128 dB (Fig. 5–10). Incoming sound is changed into electricity via the microphone located on top. When the dial is turned all the way clockwise (60 will light on the dial), the meter needle for a 50 dB sound will read at −10 dB. The needle will respond at a lower sound intensity if the C scale of the meter is used. The speed of the needle response can be switched from SLOW to FAST. A 9 volt alkaline battery makes the device portable. The meter is small and lightweight. It can be held or attached to a tripod. The microphone is most sensitive if the microphone faces the sound source.

The Radio Shack meter is not sensitive enough to indicate when optimally desirable low noise levels exist in an occupied classroom. It is sensitive

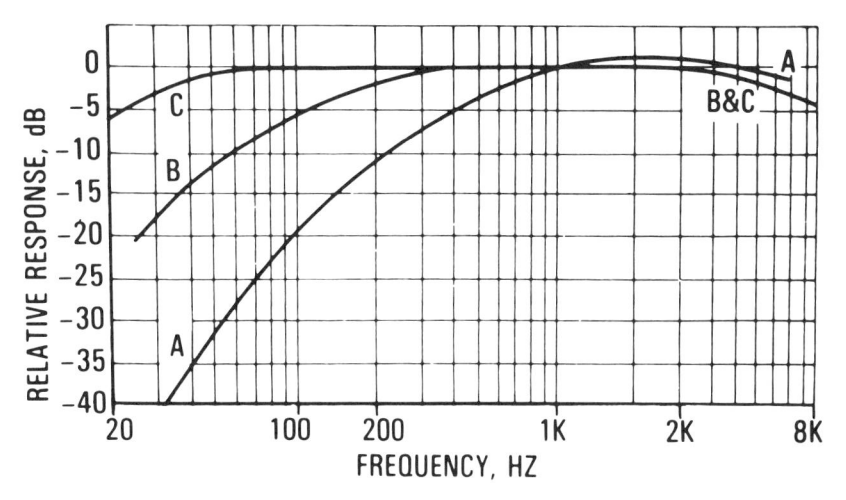

Figure 5-9. Frequency response of A, B, and C scales of a sound level meter. (From Hirschorn, M. (1982). *IAC noise control handbook* (p. F-3). Bronx, NY: Industrial Acoustics Company. Copyright 1982 by Industrial Acoustics Company. Reprinted by permission.)

102 Facilitating Classroom Listening

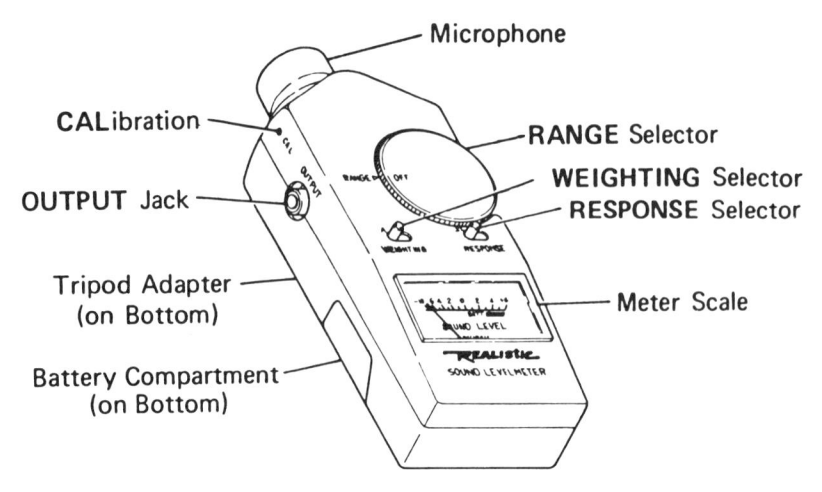

Figure 5-10. Low cost sound level meter. (From Radio Shack advertisement. Fort Worth, TX: Radio Shack, A Division of Tandy Corporation. Reprinted by permission.)

enough to indicate the equivalent of a 37 dBA measurement in an unoccupied classroom, by reading as low as 50 dBC. In an unoccupied classroom, the dBA meter indication is 13 dB lower than the dBC meter indication.

The Radio Shack meter is, however, a very practical device. It can be used to measure (1) signal intensities in decibels at various distances from a teacher and (2) noise intensities in decibels of loud background noise, fan or projector noise, people speaking, chairs being moved, books dropped, and so on. A teacher can measure (1) overall noise levels in various locations outside of a school and (2) sound intensities of students' voices and loud music from various distances.

A teacher can also estimate the RT of a classroom by use of a simple formula that incorporates the volume (V) of the room, the total absorption (A) of the room surfaces, and a constant (0.05).

$$RT = 0.05 \ V/A$$

RT is measured in seconds, V in cubic feet, and A in sabins. As indicated by the formula, the A has 20 times more influence on the RT than the V. As room dimensions (V) are increased there is a slight increase in the RT because it takes longer for the reflected sounds to reach the partitions where they can be absorbed.

The volume of the room is calculated by multiplying length × width × height in feet. Multiply by 0.05 to get a value for the numerator of the equation. Figuring the denominator of the equation is more involved.

The absorption of each room surface (ceiling, floor, four walls) is the product of the area of that surface and the absorption coefficient of the surface lining it. For the absorption coefficient, take the average of the absorption coefficients at 500, 1000, and 2000 Hz for the material in question. Sound absorption coefficients for common materials are included in Table 5–2. Add the separate absorptions for the ceiling, floor, and four walls to obtain the total absorption in sabins, which is the number placed in the denominator of the equation.

The RT in seconds is then obtained by dividing the numerator by the denominator of the equation. Following this procedure, a classroom 7 feet high, 16 feet wide and 24 feet long has a volume of 2688 cubic feet, which when multiplied by 0.05 = 134.4. If the walls are plaster on concrete, the ceiling plaster on lath, and the floor wood parquet on concrete, the absorption coefficients are 0.06, 0.05, and 0.06 respectively. The corresponding areas are: 112 square feet, 112 square feet, 168 square feet, 168 square feet, 384 square feet, and 384 square feet. The corresponding separate absorptions are: 6.72, 6.72, 10.08, 10.08, 19.2, and 23.02 sabins, respectively. The total absorption is 77.8 sabins. Divide 134.4 by 77.8 and the RT = 1.73 seconds. This very hard room results in an excessive RT.

If the walls are left as they are, but ½" acoustical tile suspended from the ceiling and carpet installed on the floor, the absorption coefficients for the ceiling and floor will increase to 0.66 and 0.37. The absorption for the ceiling and floor will correspondingly increase to 253.44 and 142.08 sabins, respectively. The total absorption will increase to 429.12 sabins. Divide 134.4 by 429.12 and the RT = 0.31 seconds. By changing the ceiling and floor from hard to soft surfaces, the reverberation characteristics of the classroom are dramatically improved. Provided noise levels can be kept low, this classroom should now provide a desirable instructional and listening environment.

After calculating RTs for a number of rooms, the teacher will be able to estimate RTs of additional rooms. Adding acoustical tile to the ceiling will reduce RT of a hard room to perhaps 0.7 seconds. Adding carpet will reduce the RT to 0.4 seconds or less. Further reduction of RT can be accomplished by acoustically treating the walls. Adding people or soft chairs to the room will reduce the RT another 0.1 seconds.

ALLEVIATION

Reducing Reverberation

Previous discussion in this chapter indicates that reducing reverberation is a matter of increasing the sound absorption of room sur-

Table 5-2. Sound Absorption Coefficients for Common Materials

Material	125	250	500	1k	2k	4k	NRC rating
Walls							
Brick	0.03	0.03	0.03	0.04	0.05	0.07	0.05
Concrete painted	0.10	0.05	0.06	0.07	0.09	0.08	0.05
Window glass	0.35	0.25	0.18	0.12	0.07	0.04	0.15
Marble	0.01	0.01	0.01	0.01	0.02	0.02	0.00
Plaster or concrete	0.12	0.09	0.07	0.05	0.05	0.04	0.05
Plywood	0.28	0.22	0.17	0.09	0.10	0.11	0.15
Concrete block, coarse	0.36	0.44	0.31	0.29	0.39	0.25	0.35
Heavyweight drapery	0.14	0.35	0.55	0.72	0.70	0.65	0.60
Fiberglass wall treatment, 1 inch (2.5 cm)	0.08	0.32	0.99	0.76	0.34	0.12	0.60
Fiberglass wall treatment, 7 inch (17.8 cm)	0.86	0.99	0.99	0.99	0.99	0.99	0.95
Wood panelling on glass fiber blanket	0.40	0.99	0.80	0.50	0.40	0.30	0.65
Floors							
Wood parquet on concrete	0.04	0.04	0.07	0.06	0.06	0.07	0.05
Linoleum	0.02	0.03	0.03	0.03	0.03	0.02	0.05
Carpet on concrete	0.02	0.06	0.14	0.37	0.60	0.65	0.30
Carpet on foam rubber padding	0.08	0.24	0.57	0.69	0.71	0.73	0.55
Ceilings							
Plaster, gypsum, or lime on lath	0.14	0.10	0.06	0.05	0.04	0.03	0.05
Acoustic tiles ⅝ inch (1/6 cm), suspended 16 inches (40.6 cm)	0.25	0.28	0.46	0.71	0.86	0.93	0.60
Acoustic tiles ½ inch (1.2 cm), suspended 16 inches (40.6 cm) from ceiling	0.52	0.37	0.50	0.69	0.79	0.78	0.60
The same as above, but cemented directly to ceiling	0.10	0.22	0.61	0.66	0.74	0.72	0.55
High absorptive panels, 1 inch (2.5 cm), suspended 16 inches (40.6 cm) from ceiling	0.58	0.88	0.75	0.99	1.00	0.96	0.90
Others							
Upholstered seats	0.19	0.37	0.56	0.67	0.61	0.59	0.55
Audience in upholstered seats	0.39	0.57	0.80	0.94	0.92	0.87	0.80
Grass	0.11	0.26	0.60	0.69	0.92	0.99	0.61
Soil	0.15	0.25	0.40	0.55	0.60	0.60	0.45
Water surface	0.01	0.01	0.01	0.02	0.02	0.03	0.00

From *Acoustics—Architectural theory and practice*. Park Ridge, IL: American Board Products Association. Copyright 1975 by American Hardboard Association. Reprinted by permission.

faces by acoustical treatment. Acoustical treatment of classrooms is usually at three levels: (1) no acoustical treatment, (2) acoustical tile on ceilings, and (3) acoustical tile on ceilings combined with carpet on floor. The walls of classrooms are seldom acoustically treated. They are left hard and nonporous like the windows certain of them include.

Untreated or hard room surfaces cause classrooms to be highly reverberant. A contributor to a book on designing learning environments recently wrote

> Buildings erected between 1915 and 1940 contained all the characteristics of poor acoustical treatment. Noticeable were high ceilings, hard walls, hard floors, parallel walls, hard ceilings, and reflective windows. The transmission of sound in these buildings left much to be desired. Sound bounced disastrously from the many reflective surfaces, creating the re-echo of an echo chamber in its distracting hollow reproductions. The instructor needed to shout in order to be heard, in which case the sounds reverberated so as to make communication unintelligible (Silverstone, 1981, p. 79).

Some highly reverberant rooms are still being used for teaching (Fig. 5-11). Their RTs vary from 1 to 3 seconds. Newer classrooms usually have acoustic ceiling, with resulting RTs of 0.6 to 0.8 seconds. Perhaps the most practical further acoustical treatment is installing inexpensive carpet, preferably padded, on a classroom floor. In combination with acoustical ceiling tile, carpet can reduce RT to 0.3 to 0.4 seconds.

By spending another $50 to 100 on a classroom, small fiberglass panels can be installed at various wall locations to break up remaining sound reflection. Owens Corning Corporation produces fiberglass panels with high absorption coefficients for less than $1 per square foot. A local building supply store should also have acoustic panels. Select colors that blend with existing room colors. Painting is not recommended, since it fills porous surfaces.

When a room is occupied, the RT is slightly less than when it is unoccupied. Also, soft chairs and other furniture will result in a slight reduction of RT. These changes, however, do not have a major impact on RT.

Some special classrooms for the hearing impaired have been built with nonparallel walls. This also reduces room reflection but is not a practical method for acoustically modifying existing rooms. Reducing room height (volume) has a minor effect on RT, as revealed through the RT formula.

Acoustical treatment can effect some sound frequencies more than others. Table 5-2 reveals differences in absorption coefficients for frequencies from 125 to 4000 Hz. Carpet, for example, particularly reduces the reverberation of the middle and high frequency sounds.

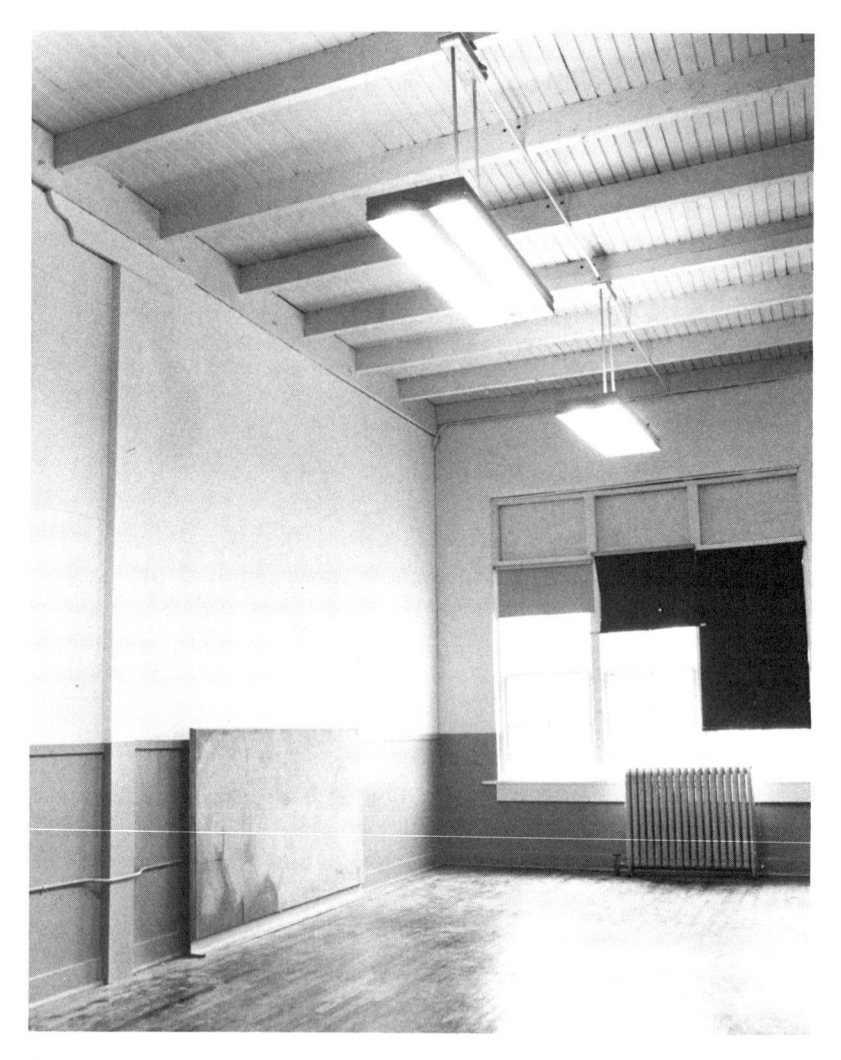

Figure 5-11. An old classroom with hard surfaces and a noisy radiator. (Courtesy of Utah State University.)

ceiling tile has a more uniform effect in reducing reverberation of various sound frequencies. Figure 5-12 shows RTs of low, middle, and high frequency sounds for two levels of acoustical treatment.

Reducing Noise

Previous discussion in this book indicates that a major noise problem exists in schools. Noise measures recently obtained from occupied classrooms in the Dallas and Chicago areas may be representative.

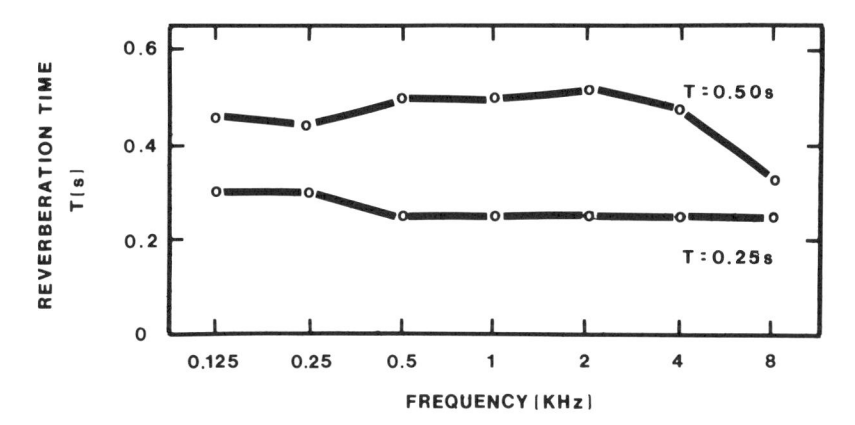

Figure 5-12. Reverberation time of a small laboratory room before and after ceilings and walls were covered with ¼" thick masonite panels. (From Nabelek, A., and Nabelek, I. (1978). Principles of noise control (p. 79). In D. Lipscomb (Ed.), *Noise and audiology*. Baltimore: University Park Press. Copyright 1978 by University Park Press. Reprinted by permission.)

Noise intensity values were acceptable in a small special classroom of a school for the hearing impaired but unacceptable in all other learning settings. The specific noise levels were as follows: 45 dBA in a small special classroom, 60 dBA in a regular traditional classroom, 60 dBA in a mainstream classroom for the hearing impaired, 70+ dBA in an open plan classroom, and 70 to 90 dBA in gymnasiums, cafeterias, and computer terminal rooms.

The school environment is filled with unwanted sound from many sources. Noise sources are outside and inside the school. Air-borne noise comes from people and equipment outside and inside the school. Structure-borne noise comes from the mechanical vibration of loose plumbing pipes and poorly supported heat and air conditioning ducts. This vibration is conducted directly through floors, ceilings, and walls of the school.

Community noise increases each year with the purchase of more and more motorized equipment. Consequently, many schools that were originally built in quiet environments are now located in noisy environments. Schools can establish policies, however, to restrict the use of motorcycles, power mowers, and similar noisy equipment to before and after school. A wall barrier can also be placed between a heavily traveled road and a nearby school (Fig. 5–13). Outside walls can be made of dense materials, doors can have solid cores, and windows can be double-paned to prevent excessive noise from entering buildings. Doors and windows to the outside need to be closed, or outside sound will be propagated into the

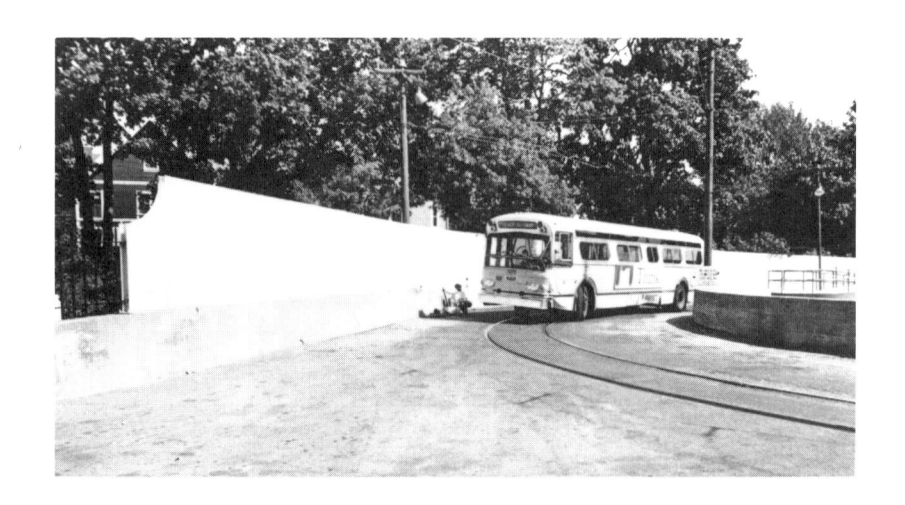

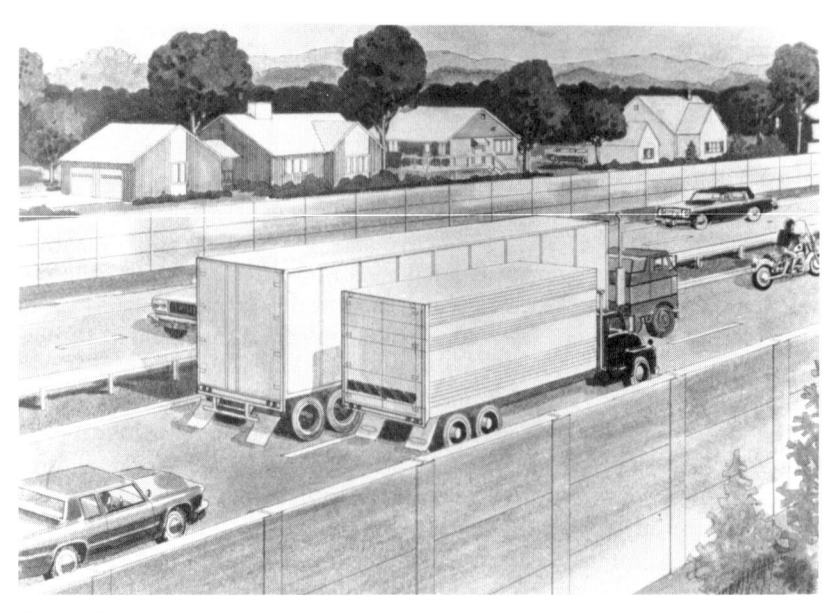

Figure 5-13. Sound absorptive steel barriers for reducing and isolating traffic noise by 15 dBA. (From Hirschorn, M. (1982). *IAC noise control handbook* (0-1, 0-3). Bronx, NY: Industrial Acoustic Company. Copyright 1982 by Industrial Acoustics Company. Reprinted by permission.)

school. Even if a small opening exists, sound will get in through direct or diffracted waves.

Intense noise is generated by equipment, teachers, and children within schools. Shop areas, computer rooms, gymnasiums, cafeterias, hallways, and even classrooms are sources of air borne sound that is transmitted into adjacent areas of school. Furnace and air conditioning rooms and rest rooms are sources of structure-borne vibrations that are conducted into other rooms. The ceilings and walls of very noisy rooms and hallways can be acoustically treated to dissipate reflected sound. Intensely noisy machines can be kept lubricated. Remaining noise from machines is best reduced by shielding it near its source with foam or fiberglass absorbent materials. When the noise strikes the absorptive material, it is converted into noiseless heat energy. Structure-borne sound can be reduced by servicing pipe and duct support structures to prevent mechanical vibration. Noisy children and teachers can be counseled to be more quiet.

Reducing noise within classrooms is of particular importance. Noise is generated both outside of and within classrooms. Classroom partitions (floor, ceiling, and walls) should be made of dense materials to keep noise out. The sound incident to the partition will be much more intense than the sound transmitted through if dense materials are used. Outside-to-inside noise reduction, called sound transmission loss (STL), will also be greater if inside partition surfaces are acoustically treated (Fig. 5-14).

The STL values at low, middle, and high frequencies for common building materials are shown in Table 5-3. A single sound transmission class (STC) rating in decibels makes it easy to compare the effectiveness of various building materials in keeping noise out. For example, solid concrete has an STC rating of 47 dB, a sealed double window 28 dB, and a solid core wood door with weather stripping 27dB.

When regular classrooms and open classrooms are occupied with a teacher and students, their noise levels typically increase 15 to 20 and 25 dBA, respectively. This noise increase comes from talking, chairs moving, books dropping, and other distractive and disruptive sounds that teachers and students produce in the classroom. In an open plan classroom, several teachers and many more children make unwanted sounds, which contributes to a substantial dBA noise increase.

In an open plan school, sounds from various sources are no longer restricted to specific learning areas but are diffused throughout wings of buildings. A comparison of traditional classroom use and open plan classroom use of the same school space is illustrated in Figure 5-15. In an open plan classroom, the 70+ dBA noise levels result in S/N ratios of −5 to −15 dB. Teachers tire their voices trying to be heard. Normal

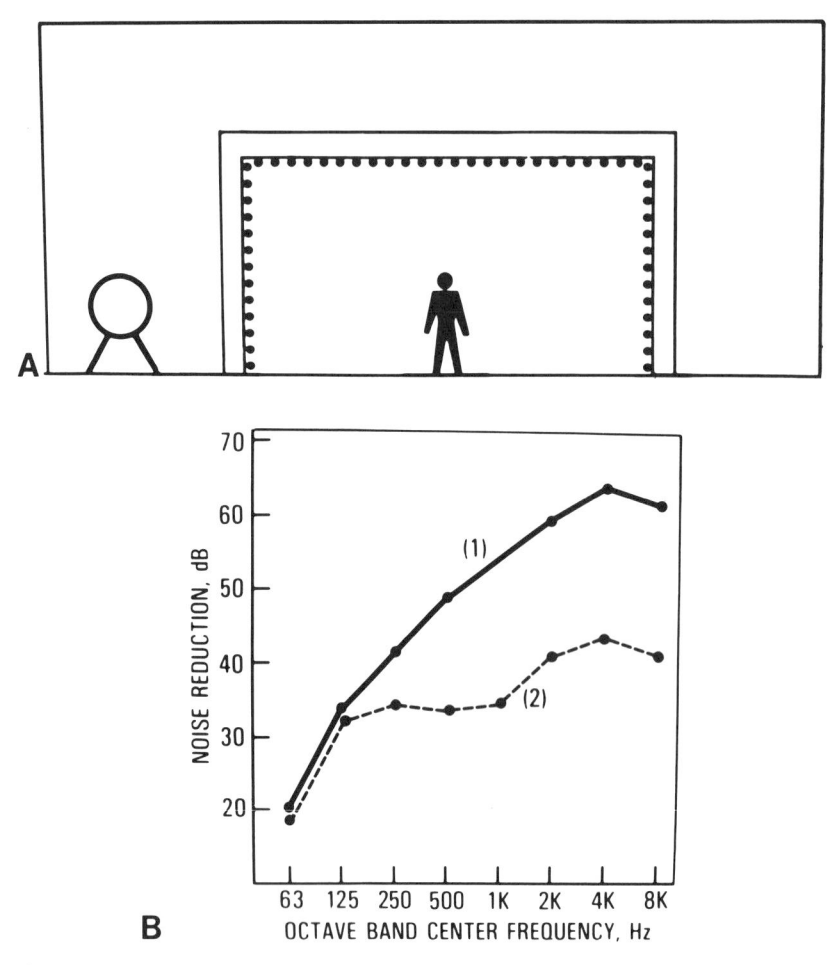

Figure 5-14. (A) An outside noise source and room. (B) The sound transmission losses in decibels of (1) highly absorptive inside room surfaces versus (2) reflective inside room surfaces. (From Hirschorn, M. (1982). *IAC noise control handbook* (D-8, D-9). Bronx, NY: Industrial Acoustics Company. Copyright 1982 by Industrial Acoustics Company. Reprinted by permission.)

hearing students strain to hear. Hard of hearing students do not detect the soft sounds of speech. Perhaps the best solution to the open plan school is to restore the traditional classroom walls and specific learning spaces.

In summary, reducing noise should take place outside a school, inside all areas of a school, and inside classrooms. Both air-borne sound

Table 5-3. Sound Transmission Loss (STL) and Sound Transmission Class (STC) Ratings in dB for Common Building Materials

Material	Total thickness inch	Total thickness cm	125	250	500	Frequency (Hz) 1k	2k	4k	STC rating
Walls									
Solid concrete	3	8	35	40	44	52	59	64	47
Concrete (6;15), layers of plaster	7	18	39	42	50	58	64	66	53
Solid concrete blocks, layers of paster	16	41	50	54	59	65	71	68	63
Brick (4½;11), layers of plaster	5½	14	34	34	41	50	56	58	42
Brick (9;23), layers of plaster	10	25	41	43	49	55	57	59	52
Stone (24;61), layers of plaster	25	64	50	53	52	58	61	68	56
Hollow concrete block	6	15	32	33	40	48	51	48	43
Cinder block (4;10), layers of plaster	5¼	13	36	37	44	51	55	62	46
Hollow gypsum block (3;8), layers of plaster	4	10	39	34	38	43	48	46	40
Double brick (4½;11) wall, cavity (2;5), layer of plaster	12	31	37	41	48	60	60	61	49
Double brick (4½;11) wall, cavity (6;15), layer of plaster	18	46	48	54	58	64	69	75	62
Solid sanded gypsum plaster	2	5	36	28	35	39	48	52	36
Solid gypsum core moveable partition	2¼	6	34	34	37	38	39	45	36
Floor-ceiling									
Reinforced concrete slab	4	10	48	42	45	55	57	66	44
Reinforced concrete as above + carpeting and pad	4½	11	48	42	45	55	57	66	44
Concrete (4½;11), wood flooring, layer of plaster	7	18	35	37	42	49	58	62	46
Concrete (4⅝;11), screed, suspended plaster ceiling	10	25	38	41	45	52	57	59	48
Concrete (6;15), wood, battens floating on glass wool, layer of plaster	9½	24	38	44	52	55	60	65	55
Wooden joists (8;20), floor gypsum wallboard	9½	24	19	24	31	35	45	42	34
Wooden joists (7;18), wood + linoleum, reeds + plaster	9½	24	24	27	35	44	52	58	39
Windows									
Double window	⅜	1.0	21	22	19	24	25	33	24
Double window sealed	⅜	1.0	20	25	20	30	34	34	28
Double window with cracks	⅜	1.0	18	21	19	20	22	30	20
Doors									
Solid core wood, weather strip	1¾	4.0	21	27	30	26	25	29	27
Hollow core wood, weather strip	1¾	4.0	14	15	17	18	22	29	20

From *Principles of noise control*. In D. Lipscomb (Ed.). *Noise and audiology*. Baltimore, University Park Press. Copyright 1978 by University Park Press. Reprinted by permission.

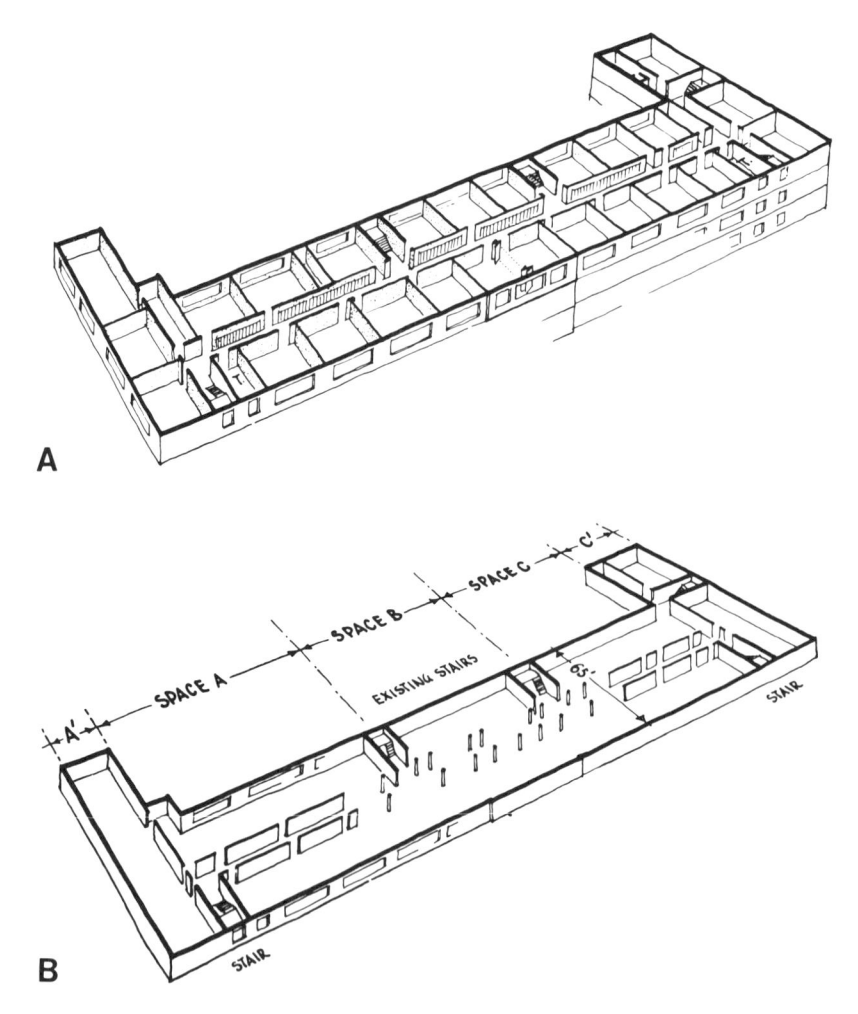

Figure 5-15. School space with (A) and without (B) classroom partitions. (From Leggett, S., et al. (1977). *Planning flexible learning spaces* (p. 88). New York: McGraw-Hill. Copyright 1977 by McGraw-Hill Book Company. Reprinted by permission.)

and structure-borne noise needs to be reduced. Noise should be controlled at its sources, kept from being transmitted into or through a school building, and absorbed by acoustical treatment. Teachers and students should be encouraged to be quieter. Open plan classrooms should be eliminated, in light of their devastating effect upon listening.

Acoustical Control Plan

Reducing reverberation and noise in a school benefits teachers and students, especially students with special listening needs. An acoustical control plan (ACP) should be developed for each school. This plan should be like an individualized educational plan (IEP) for a handicapped child. The school might be considered to be handicapped acoustically, deleteriously affecting all teachers and students. The ACP should describe current reverberation and noise levels, general and specific objectives, persons responsible for implementing the plan, and evaluation procedures. A study team should be appointed to write the ACP. The school principal should be the team director. Other team members might include an educational audiologist or speech-language pathologist, teacher representatives, student representatives, a custodian, a business manager, and a consulting acoustical engineer.

The ACP should be based on reverberation and noise data. A member of the school staff, preferably the audiologist or speech-language pathologist, can be given responsibility for obtaining this information. The RT formula and absorption table can be used to obtain reverberation data on each classroom and other learning area in the school. An inexpensive sound level meter can be used to secure noise source and level data. Optionally, more exacting RT and noise data can be obtained from the acoustical engineer, using more sophisticated equipment, provided funds are available.

The data collector can walk throughout the school environment and surrounding area, stopping to listen to and list noise sources. At the same time, dBA values of noise can be measured and recorded. These measures can be taken near noise sources and at each site where teaching, learning, and speaker-listener interaction occurs. This inspection and measurement program should be conducted as many times as necessary to account for noise variations during the school day and school week.

The ACP program should be implemented vigorously and evaluated carefully. The entire school staff and student body should participate. Short-range and long-range effects should be met on schedule. Heretofore, the educational establishment has not conducted a systematic program of reverberation and noise reduction. Implementing acoustical change in the schools will be a challenging but rewarding undertaking.

SUMMARY

Undesirable room acoustics are commonplace in the schools of the nation. Students with normal hearing and especially hard of hearing students have difficulty listening. Reverberation is excessive, smearing

114 Facilitating Classroom Listening

the speech of the teacher. Noise is too intense, masking the speech of the teacher. Simple procedures are described for obtaining reverberation and noise levels in school. An Acoustical Control Plan for reducing room reverberation and school noise is discussed.

FURTHER READINGS

The *Noise Control Reference Handbook* (Industrial Acoustics Company, Bronx, NY, 1982) by Martin Hirschorn is a rich source of basic and practical information on sound propagation and room acoustics. Product literature, equipment and materials, and consultive assistance are available from the IAC. Anna and Igor Nabelek's chapter on principles of noise control in David Lipscomb's book *Noise in Audiology* (University Park Press, Baltimore, 1978) provides additional needed source material. Their chapter on room acoustics and speech perception in Jack Katz's book *Handbook of Clinical Audiology* (Williams & Wilkins, Baltimore, 1985) extends this information. The chapter by Terese Finitzo-Hieber on classroom acoustics in Ross Roeser and Marion Down's book *Auditory Disorders in School Children* (Thieme-Stratton, New York, 1981) describes how the combination of reverberation and noise makes learning a more difficult task. Ann Wilson-Vlotman's chapter on management and coordination of services in the book *Educational Audiology for the Hard of Hearing Child,* by Frederick Berg, James Blair, Steven Viewhweg, and Ann Wilson-Vlotman, is important source material for facilitating educational change in the school.

APPENDIX

Audiometric Room

Audiometric rooms can be located or installed within school buildings. They are constructed of materials that assure controlled sound environment, including a sound-proof ventilating system. Figure 5–16 shows single and multiple occupancy units and a ventilation silencer. The silencer provides complete or partial noise control and permits air flow. The single occupancy unit is portable, has a single wall, and may be on casters. The multiple occupancy unit is more permanent and can be of single or double wall construction. It may rest directly on the building floor or on vibration insulators. Vibration insulators keep out structure-borne sound, which is caused by direct mechanical contact with a sound source. The NRC (absorption coefficient) rating of the walls is a mini-

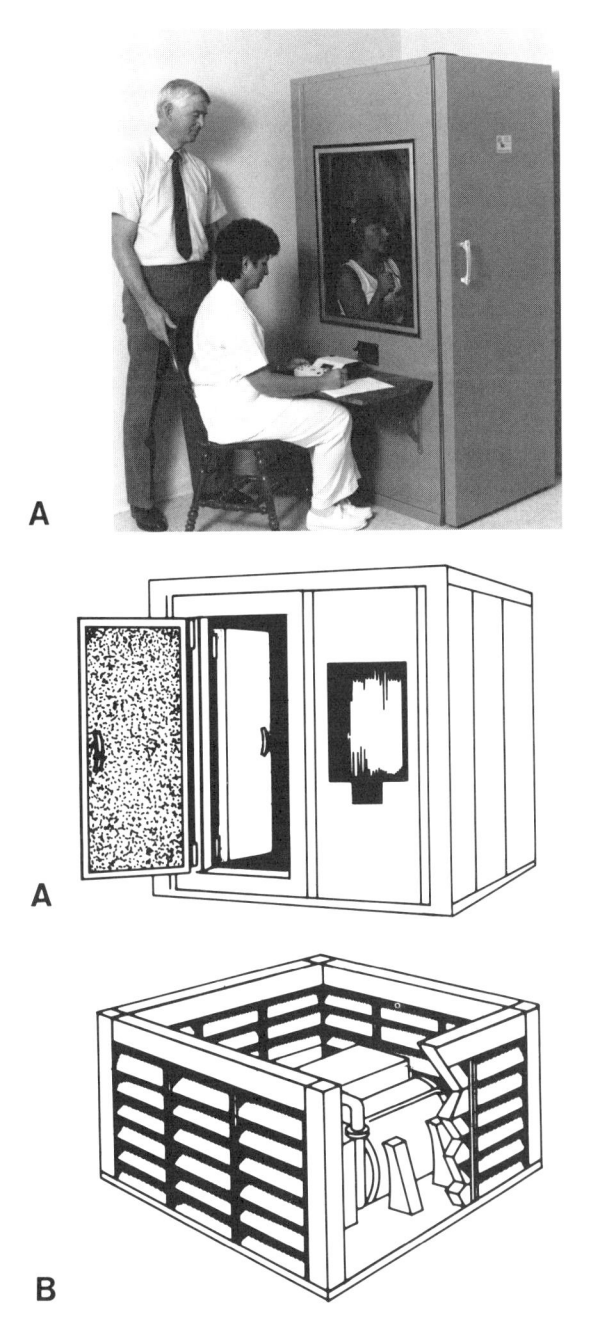

Figure 5-16. Sound shelters (A) and ventilation silencer (B). (From Hirschorn, M. (1982). *IAC noise control handbook* (K-4). Bronx, NY: Industrial Acoustics Company. Copyright 1982 by Industrial Acoustics Company. Reprinted by permission.)

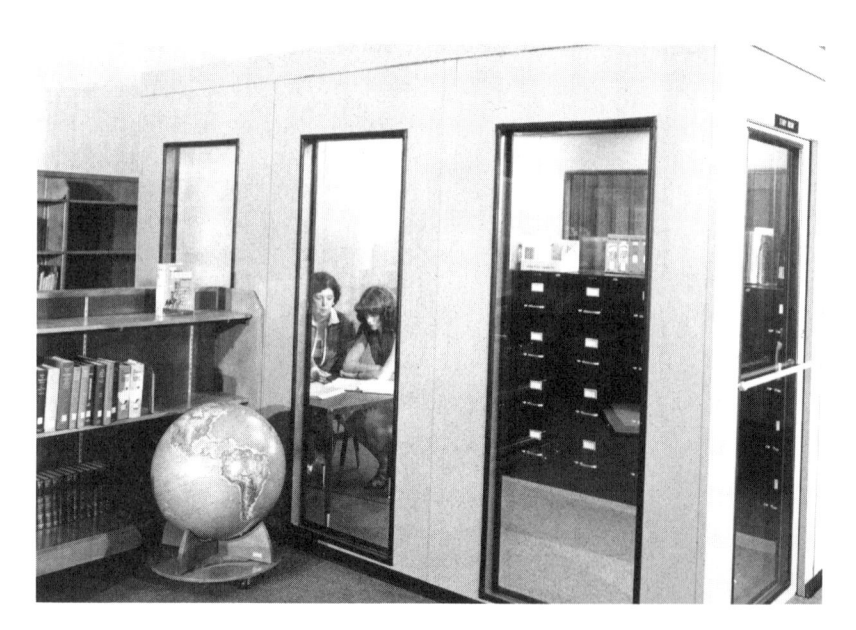

Figure 5-17. Educational study rooms that provide acoustical privacy, a well-illuminated environment and soundproof ventilation for teaching, testing, conferences, or study. (From Hirschorn, M. (1982). *IAC noise control handbook* (K-4). Bronx, NY: Industrial Acoustics Company. Copyright 1982 by Industrial Acoustics Company. Reprinted by permission.

mum of 0.95. Permissible outside air-borne noise levels are minimally 70dBA.

Educational Study Room

A space within a classroom in school can be enclosed and acoustically isolated. Figure 5-17 shows educational study rooms that are specially constructed to provide 45 dBA outside-to-inside STC and 61 dB room-to-room STC. Double paned windows separated by a layer of air and noise-lock doors are included.

Chapter 6

Hearing Aids

CASE STUDY

KB is a 12 year old girl in the sixth grade. She has a high tone sensorineural bilateral hearing loss. The degree and configuration of hearing loss in both ears is about the same. Her audiograms slope downward gradually, from 30 to 35 dB at 125 Hz to 70 to 75 dB at 8000 Hz. Her average loss in the left ear is 50 dB and in the right ear 55 dB.

KB has learning, social, and emotional problems. Her academic achievement test scores reveal that she has been behind her peers in school and that her academic deficit has increased with time in school. Currently, her average achievement scores are typical of fourth grade children. She is further behind in vocabulary and paragraph meaning than in spelling and arithmetic computations.

A community psychologist has administered the Weschler Intelligence Scale for Children, Revised Scale (WISC-R) to KB. Her scores for verbal subtests were substantially lower than normal. Her scores for the performance subtests were within normal limits.

The speech-language pathologist has administered vocabulary, language, and word recognition tests to KB. Her scores reveal low verbal comprehension, low reading comprehension, depressed auditory skills, and fair lipreading skills.

KB's teachers have reported that she is socially withdrawn and often excluded from peer activities. She appears to have a low self image. Her parents have become increasingly concerned about KB's educational, social, and emotional problems.

KB's hearing loss appears to be congenital. However, it was not diagnosed until she was 4 years old. At that time she was tested by an audiologist and seen by an otologist, both of whom recommended amplification. KB's parents took her to a local hearing aid dispenser, who made ear impressions for her. She was fitted with binaural behind-the-ear (BTE) hearing aids. However, the dispenser spent little time assisting KB to learn to use the aids optimally. Sometimes KB would wear two aids, sometimes one aid, and sometimes no aid at all.

When KB began school, her parents took her to another audiologist, who found that the aids needed service and that KB needed new earmolds. Since then, KB has more willingly worn hearing aids. She has had three sets of hearing aids during the last 8 years. Still, her parents report that keeping the aids on KB and keeping them working well has been a struggle. There has been a continuing concern that KB has not obtained optimal benefit from the aids.

KB's teachers have been told to provide her with preferential seating. They have been asked to encourage her to sit toward the front of the room so she can hear and lipread better. Some teachers have followed these directions and others have not. KB herself has tended to want to sit in the back of the room so she will not be noticed. She often misunderstands her teachers but does not want to be singled out for help.

KB needs systematic assistance with her hearing aids. The response of the aids should be appropriate for her hearing loss. The earmolds should be kept clean. The batteries should be checked daily. Visual inspection of the aids should be made. Daily listening checks should be made. The physical characteristics of the aids should be checked periodically. The teachers need to know how to work with KB and her parents in maintaining the aids so they work well. Service from local specialists and from the manufacturer of the aids needs to be assured.

The local school district is small and does not employ an educational audiologist. The speech-language pathologist has responsibility for hearing aids in the district. She relies on an audiologist in private practice for assistance. The audiologist fit KB with her last hearing aids.

BASIC CONSIDERATIONS

Introduction to Hearing Aids

A modern hearing aid is a miniaturized device that partially compensates for hearing loss. The aid reconfigures and amplifies sounds so a hearing impaired person can detect them more fully. The aid is attached to an earmold that delivers the reconstituted sound into an ear. One aid and mold constitute a monaural amplification system. Two aids and molds make up a binaural amplification system. A binaural hearing aid is ordinarily preferable to a monaural hearing aid.

A hearing aid can also be built to compress intensity differences in decibels between ordinarily loud and soft speech sounds. Compression amplification helps hearing impaired persons who have narrow ranges between thresholds of detection and thresholds of discomfort.

Earmolds are also fashioned to reconfigure sound to compensate for slope of hearing los. Low, middle, or high frequencies can be emphasized or suppressed by various earmold modifications.

The basic amplification function of a hearing aid causes the user to detect sounds at lower decibel levels. Aided and unaided audiograms are shown in Figure 6-1. The aid does not elevate hearing to 0 dB but does cause dramatic rise of detection thresholds.

A volume control is located on a hearing aid to adjust amplification to a desirable amount for the user. A battery is located in the aid to power the electrical circuits. A microphone picks up and changes incoming sound signals into electrical signals. An amplifier increases the amplitude

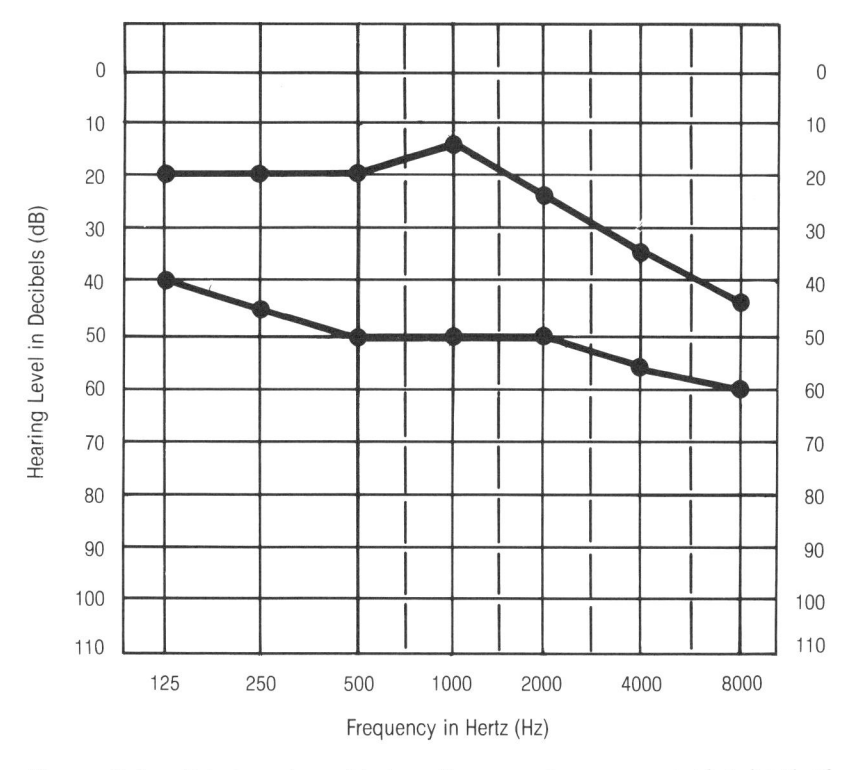

Figure 6-1. Aided and unaided audiograms for one ear of a hard of hearing student.

120 Facilitating Classroom Listening

Sound enters the aid and is picked up by the **microphone**.

Loudness can be adjusted by using the **volume control**.

The **amplifier** makes electrical power.

Battery supplies electrical power.

The **speaker** or receiver sends sound into a clear plastic tube.

The amplified sound is channeled into the ear canal

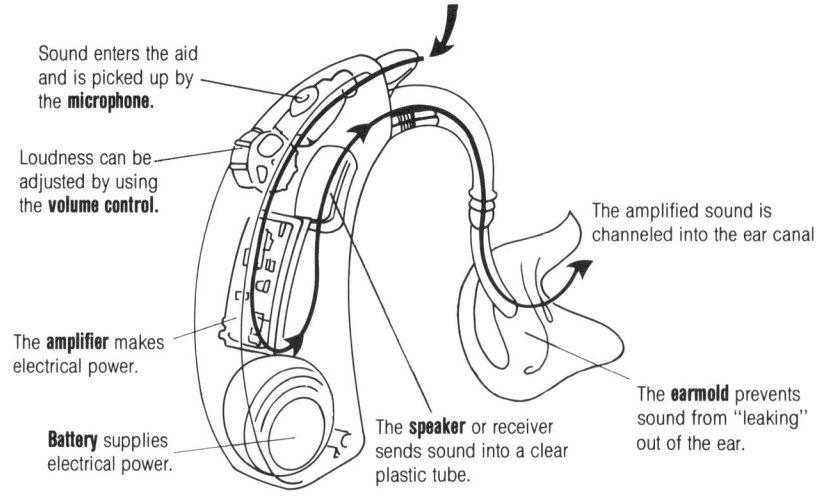

The **earmold** prevents sound from "leaking" out of the ear.

Figure 6-2. A close up look of a behind-the-ear (BTE) hearing aid and some of its component parts. From Kweskin, S., Rother, S., and McMahon, S. (1984). *Hearing aids. A guide to their wear and care* (p. 8). Daly City, CA: Patient Information Library. Copyright 1981, 1983, and 1984 by Krames Communications. Reprinted by permission.

of these signals. A speaker or receiver converts the electrical signal back into a sound signal. The amplified sound is channeled through the earmold into the ear canal. Figure 6–2 shows these hearing aid components. Other components are included in a hearing aid to reconfigure and compress amplified electrical signals.

Types of Hearing Aids

There are four hearing aid styles: behind-the-ear (BTE), in-the-ear (ITE), eyeglasses, and body (Figure 6–3). ITE aids are most commonly used by adults and BTE aids by children. Body and eyeglass aids are seldom purchased any more. Little industry effort is going into improving the body and eyeglass aids. Each of four styles of aids can now provide sufficient amplification for a child with a hearing loss as great as 90 dB. Except for the ITE aid, each style can provide 70+ dB of amplification, more than sufficient for any degree of hearing loss.

Perhaps the main reason BTE aids are recommended for children is that they can be used effectively with FM radio equipment, which bypasses noise and reverberation. ITE aids are just beginning to be used with FM equipment. A technology, effectively coupling an FM radio signal into the relatively small ITE aid, however, may be developed.

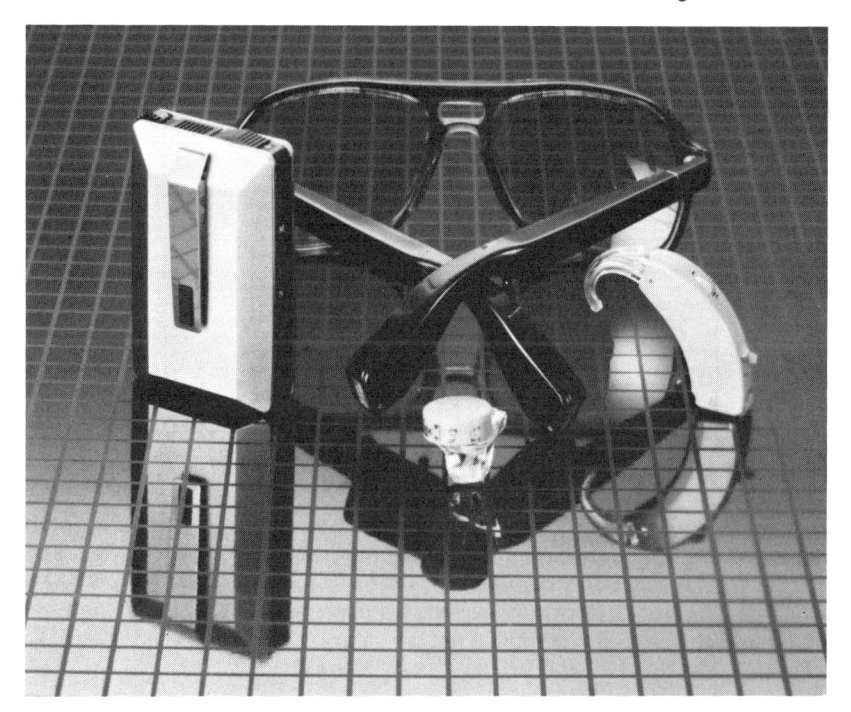

Figure 6-3. Four hearing aid styles: body, eyeglass, modular in-the-ear (ITE), and behind-the-ear (BTE). From Widex advertisement. Long Island, NY: Widex Hearing Aid Company. Reprinted by permission.

The largeness of the BTE as compared with the ITE aid enables more controls and components to be built into it. Both styles of aids have volume controls. Each can be built to reconfigure and compress incoming sound. The ITE aid can be built to have a few screwdriver controls. The BTE aid can be designed to have as many as six screwdriver controls, giving it greater adjustment versatility.

There are advantages of ITE aids, however, that may dramatically increase their use among children. First, children are sensitive about cosmetic appearance. Teenagers are especially concerned about looking "different." The ITE aid is less visible, particularly if recessed into the ear canal. Many children who refuse to wear a BTE aid may be willing to use an ITE aid. Second, factory turnaround time for replacing an outgrown ITE shell is as little as 3 days. Third, ITE aids are capable of delivering sound to the ear with characteristics more like an ideal signal than a BTE aid may be able to deliver. The main reason for this is that the ITE aid has its microphone located where the ear normally

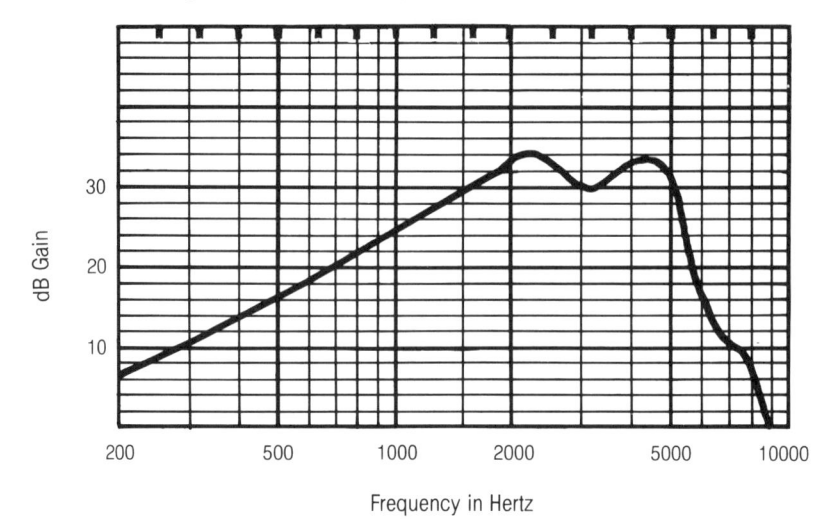

Figure 6-4. Frequency response of an in-the-ear (ITE) aid. From Wernick, J. (1980). Modular ITE hearing aids—A new generation of ITEs. *Hearing Instruments, 31,* 14. Copyright 1980 by Harcourt Brace Jovanovich. Reprinted by permission.

receives sound. This enhances high frequency sounds, provides information about directionality, and improves the detection of the signal in noise. Fourth, ITE aids often have a broader frequency response than the BTE aids. The broader the frequency response, the more sound cues are available, and the higher the listening score. Figure 6-4 shows the broad frequency response of an ITE aid. The considerable amplification at 5000 Hz helps in detecting high frequency consonant sounds like /s/ and /z/.

The direct sound input of the ITE is contrasted with the cumbersome sound input of the BTE aid in Figure 6-5. With the BTE aid, an earhook and tubing are needed to deliver output sound from the aid to the earmold and ear canal. The sound output of the ITE aid, in contrast, is already in the ear canal. The earhook and tubing present additional fitting and servicing problems.

Candidates for Hearing Aids

A child with a bilateral hearing loss of 15+ dB is a candidate for a hearing aid. This statement, however, needs to be qualified. The more permanent the loss, the greater the need for an aid. Also, the younger the

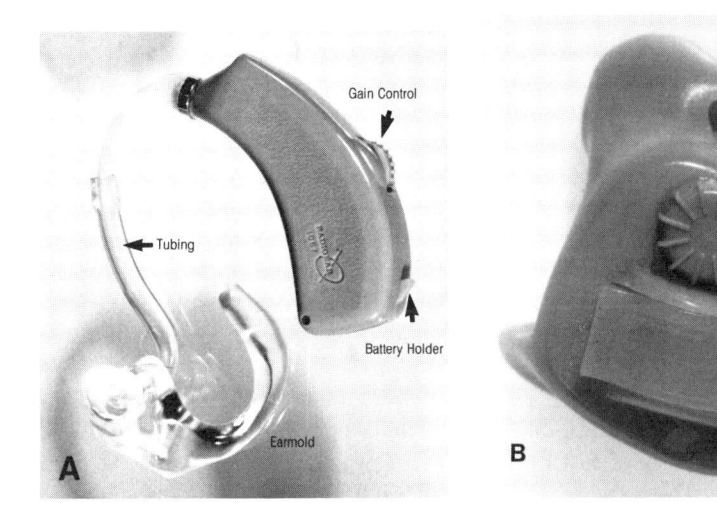

Figure 6-5. Behind-the-ear (A) and in-the-ear (B) personal amplification systems. From Lybarger, S. (1985). The physical and electroacoustic characteristics of hearing aids. In J. Katz (Ed.), *Handbook of clinical audiology* (pp. 850, 852). Baltimore: Williams & Wilkins. Copyright 1985 by Williams & Wilkins.

child, the greater the need for an aid. A child needs an aid more than an adult because the adult has already learned speech, listening, and language skills. The adult with a bilateral hearing loss as great as 40 dB may be able to "get by" without an aid. Children, in contrast, are in the process of acquiring communication skills, learning vocabulary, and acquiring verbal-cognitive skills. A normal amount of language and substantive information is not stored in their brains for filling in what they cannot hear.

When children begin school, they need to be able to hear as well as possible. Young children in school spend nearly half of their time listening. It is very important that students be able to hear teachers. Much of the time, however, the teacher-student distance averages 12 feet. At this distance, the teacher's voice is less than 60 dBA. At the same time, the noise level in the room is 60+ dBA. The negative S/N ratio results in the masking of consonants by room noise. Classrooms are also typically reverberant, so that reflected sound smears the softer sounds. The smearing of speech by reverberation cannot be alleviated with a hearing aid, but the masking of speech by noise can be relieved. The hearing aid will increase the signal level to perhaps 70 dBA so that all consonants can be detected.

Children with 25 dB bilateral hearing losses are even more in need of hearing aids. When listening at a distance, particularly in noisy and reverberant rooms, such children miss hearing some of the loud speech sounds as well as soft speech sounds. The loud speech sounds are vowels, which carry intonation and stress information critical to speech communication.

Children with 46+ dB unilateral losses also need hearing aids. They miss detecting many speech sounds when they do not wear hearing aids, particularly when the teacher faces their impaired ears while speaking. Even when the teacher faces the good ears of children with unilateral loss, these children fail to detect all of the speech sounds in noisy environments.

An option to hearing aids for school children with lesser degrees of hearing loss is the use of FM equipment which will be discussed fully in Chapter 7. Personal FM functionally brings the teacher's voice as close as 6 inches from the student's ear. Sound field FM functionally decreases the teacher-student distance to perhaps 4 feet. These FM adjustments provide students with +25 dB S/N ratios and +12 dB S/N ratios, respectively. The improvements in S/N ratios are accompanied by some relief from the smearing effects of room reverberation. Consequently, significant improvement in detection of speech sounds occurs.

Children with 40+ dB bilateral hearing loss require hearing aids whether they have access to FM equipment or not. These are the children in the regular schools who typically wear hearing aids. In schools for the deaf, where children average 90+ dB bilateral hearing loss, hearing aids are still typically worn. Whenever room acoustics are unacceptable, FM equipment is recommended, together with hearing aids for children with 40+ dB bilateral hearing loss.

Gain of Aid

The basic amplification of a hearing aid is referred to as the gain of the aid. The gain can be from 0 dB to as high as 70 dB. Low gain aids provide 40 dB of amplification, moderate gain aids 55 dB, and high gain aids 70 dB. The gain aid selected depends on the degree of detection loss of the hearing impaired person.

For practical reasons, the audiologist adjusts the gain (volume control) of the hearing aid so that incoming sound is heard at a comfortable loudness level. If the incoming sound is 65 dB, and the wearer's discomfort level is 100 dB, the gain of the aid should not be more than 35 dB or the sound output will exceed the discomfort level.

A 30 dB gain is perhaps as much detection improvement as can be expected with a 50 dB detection loss. Even with this gain, the hearing aid may make the sound uncomfortably loud, and the gain may need to be reduced somewhat. A person with a conductive hearing loss can tolerate perhaps 10 dB more gain or amplification than a person with a sensorineural hearing loss. When sound is amplified too much, it becomes distorted by the ear of the user. The percentage of sound that is understood is correspondingly reduced.

A hearing impaired person still has a detection loss when wearing an aid, but the loss is not as great as when the aid is not worn. The individual described earlier with a 50 dB unaided detection loss, for example, has an aided detection loss of 20 dB when the aid provides 30 dB of amplification. A 20 dB detection loss still seriously impairs the user's listening ability, particularly in the classroom.

Another factor limiting the usable gain of a hearing aid is acoustic feedback, or sound oscillation, heard as squeal. This occurs when the sound intensity input in dB plus the gain in dB results in an intense enough sound output in dB to cause leakage of sound back into the microphone of the aid. This leakage often occurs because the earmold of the aid does not fit well in the ear canal of the user.

When a hearing aid user talks or chews, mandibular (lower jaw) movements are accompanied by movements of the ear canal. In the past, earmolds have not been flexible enough to fill in the tiny spaces resulting from these movements. Consequently, sound leakage and squeal would occur. The newer earmolds are made of more flexible silicon material that enables the gain of the hearing aid to be turned higher before sound leakage occurs. Other techniques are also being used to enable an aid to deliver more usable gain.

It is particularly important for a hearing aid to deliver high gain to a user with a profound hearing loss. If a student has a high tone 95 dB bilateral loss, for example, the gain of a hearing aid might need to be 60 dB, or even higher, for that person to hear high frequency consonants. This is because (1) the detection loss may be 105 dB for the high frequency sounds and (2) the consonant sounds are relatively faint. The sound intensities of incoming vowels might be 65 dB, while the sound intensities of the incoming high frequency consonants might be no higher than 45 dB. This means soft sounds will need to be amplified 60+ dB to be detected.

Aided detection losses are another reason FM equipment should be used in school in addition to hearing aids. FM equipment enables a higher signal intensity in decibels to be delivered to the hearing aid. At a 12 foot teacher-student distance, the teacher's voice might have an intensity of 55 dB without FM, and 80 dB and 67 dB with personal and sound field FM, respectively. If the signal input to the hearing aid can be increased, the aid does not have to have as much gain for sound to be heard. The use of FM has the functional effect of moving the teacher much closer to the hearing impaired student.

Compression and Output Controls

Speech and environmental sounds of all intensities enter a hearing aid. Only the more intense of these, however, are detected by the user. Faint or distant sounds are masked by background noise. Vowels and consonants of conversational speech are typically heard. Loud speech and environmental sounds tend to be heard in a distorted way.

For speech communication, it would be desirable if a hearing aid could enable a user to detect all the consonants and vowels of faint, moderate, and loud speech. This would be compressing a wide intensity range of incoming sounds into a narrow range of hearing (output of aid) between the user's hearing threshold and discomfort threshold (Fig. 6-6).

A hearing aid with a compression control can partially reach this goal. It can compress a 50 to 100 dB range of incoming sound intensities into various output ranges (Fig. 6-7). An audiologist presets a compression control to a user's hearing.

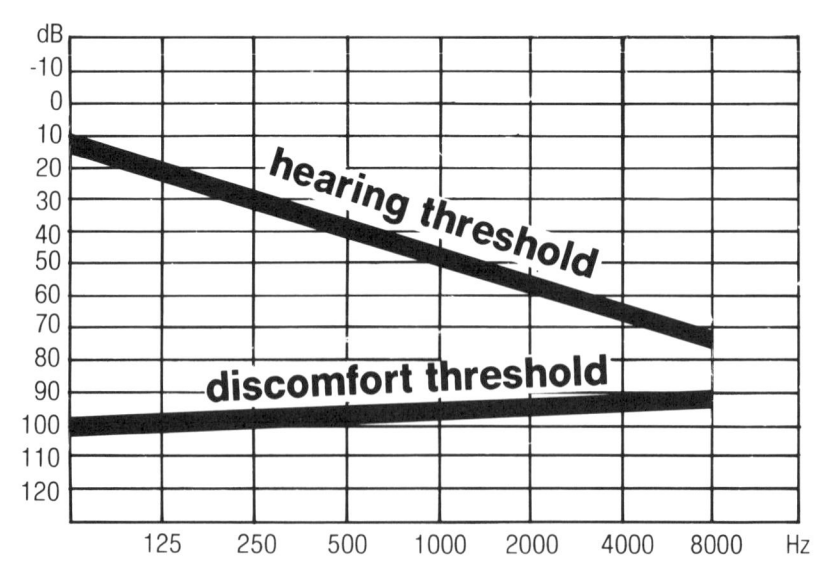

Figure 6-6. Restricted hearing area of hearing aid user. From Phillips hearing aid manual. Spring Valley, NY: Phillips Audionics Corporation. Reprinted by permission.

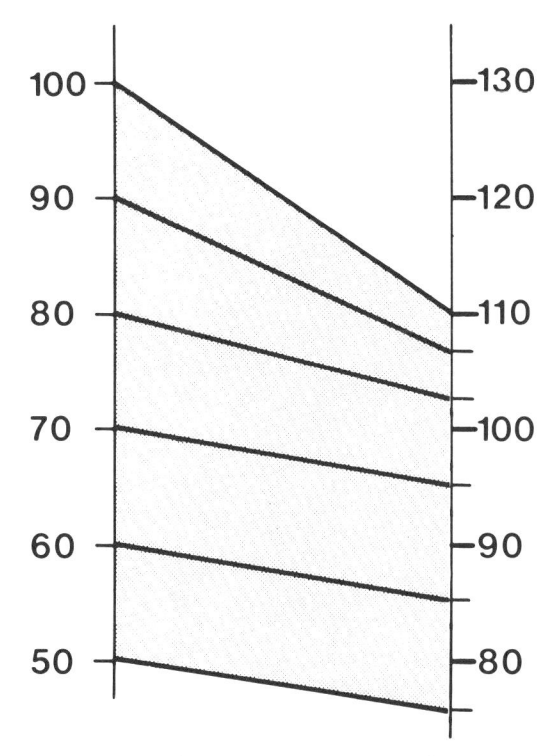

Figure 6-7. One of many input-output compression ranges in a hearing aid. From Phillips hearing aid manual. Spring Valley, NY: Phillips Audionics Corporation. Reprinted by permission.

An output control can also be built into a hearing aid. This control is adjusted by an audiologist so that sound coming out of the aid stays below a user's discomfort threshold. Output ranges vary among hearing aids. A range between 103 and 123 dB is illustrated in Figure 6-8.

Hearing aids for persons with slight or mild hearing losses and high discomfort levels do not need to be equipped with either compression or output controls. The audiologist should measure detection and discomfort thresholds to determine the need for compression and output controls. Children with sensorineural hearing impairment tend to need compression and output controls more than those with conductive hearing losses.

Frequency Adjustments

Hearing aids are built to compensate for detection loss at various frequencies. Unitron Industries, for example, produces aids for flat or sloping,

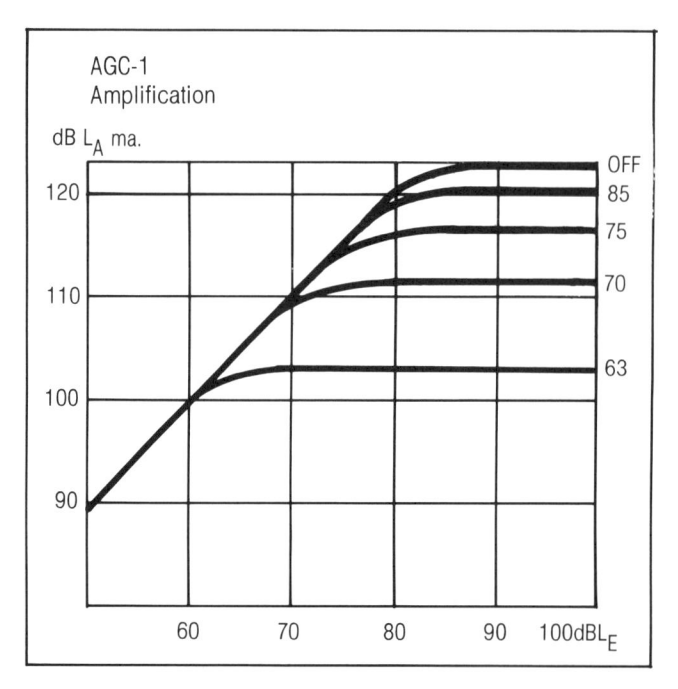

Figure 6-8. Output in decibels (vertical axis) related to input in decibels (horizontal axis) for five output control settings of a hearing aid. From Bernafon hearing aid advertisement booklet. Mountainside, NY: Bernafon. Reprinted by permission.

low frequency (reverse slope), and high frequency losses. Their fitting guide is shown in Figure 6-9.

Many hearing aids are also equipped with one or two tone controls for frequency adjustment. A low tone control varies the amplification of low frequency sounds. A high tone control varies the amplification of high frequencies. The audiologist presets these controls to the audiogram configuration (Fig. 6-10).

Earmolds of BTE aids are also fashioned and modified to compensate for various slopes of detection loss. Various vents are drilled in earmolds to suppress low frequency amplification. Damping elements are used to reduce middle frequency peaks. Sound bore changes, such as a horn effect, are used to enhance high frequency amplification. Figure 6-11 shows the frequencies affected for each of these three types of earmold modification. Similar modifications are made in ITE shells.

Earmolds and Shells

Earmolds and shells also function to keep hearing aids stationary. Earmolds anchor BTE aids; shells house ITE aids.

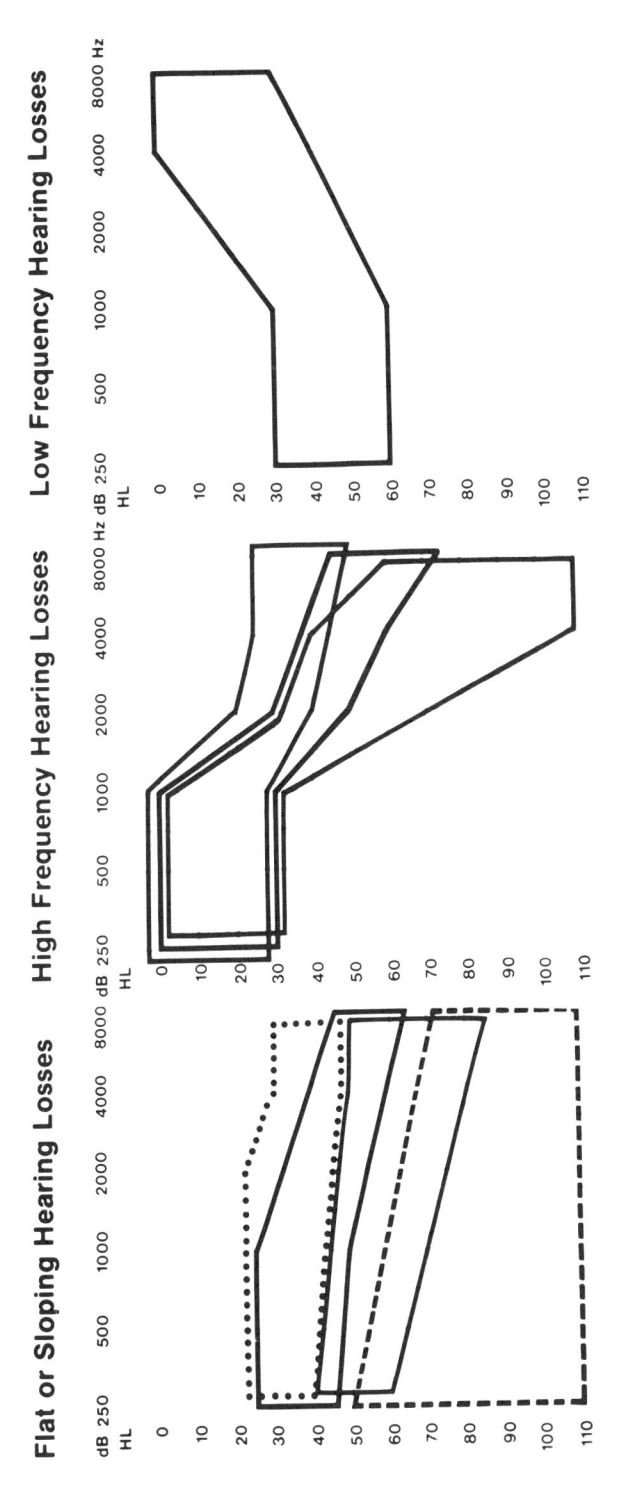

Figure 6-9. Fitting guide for hearing aids according to various hearing loss configurations. From Unitron technical summary and fitting guide. Port Huron, MI: Unitron Industries. Reprinted by permission.

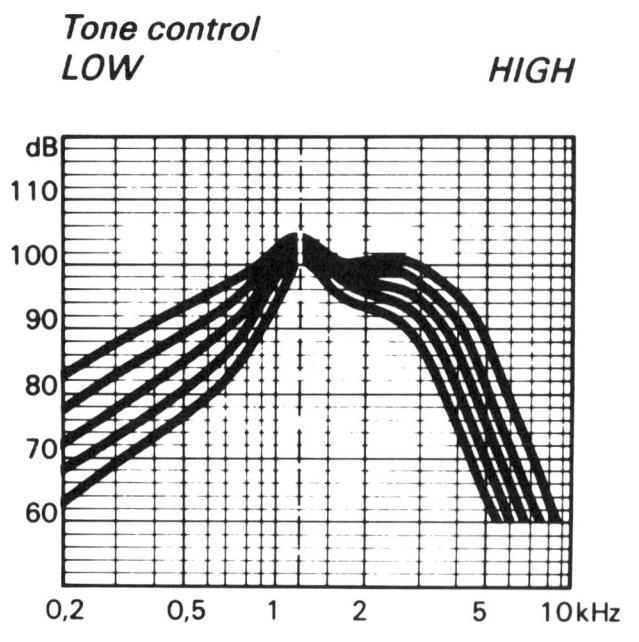

Figure 6-10. The effects of low and high tone adjustments on hearing aid frequency response. From Bernafon hearing aid advertisement booklet. Mountainside, NJ: Bernafon. Reprinted by permission.

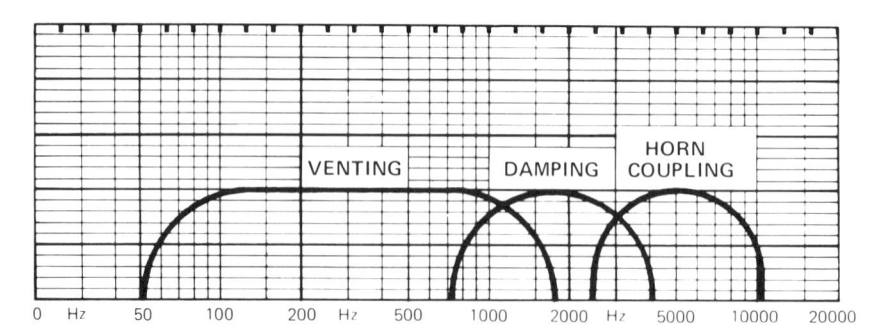

Figure 6-11. Frequencies modified by venting, damping, and sound bore changes in earmolds. From Staab, W. (1982). Earmold acoustics hearing aid systems fittings. *Audiotone Technical Reports, 3,* 1. Phoenix: Audiotone. A Division of Lear Siegler. Reprinted by permission.

Earmolds of BTE aids and shells of ITE aids are made in earmold laboratories from impressions of ears. An audiologist can make an impression of a person's ear in less than 15 minutes. The same impression is used to make any style of mold or shell requested. Ordinarily, the less the hearing loss, the less the material needed for an earmold.

A shell (full) mold is needed for a child with a severe or profound hearing loss who uses a BTE aid. This reduces the likelihood of acoustic feedback and resultant squeal. A full-concha shell is used if an ITE aid is used. This enables more features to be included in the aid and increases the likelihood it can be used with FM equipment.

Shells for ITE aids and some molds for BTE aids are made with a hard material. Many molds for BTE aids are made of a softer, more pliable material. Ordinarily, a softer material is selected for the ear of a child using a BTE aid.

Binaural and Monaural Fittings

Children are usually fitted with two aids (binaural) rather than one aid (monaural). Children with both ears impaired appear to perform better communicatively, socially, and academically when using two aids rather than one. The two aids need to be matched so that sound is heard equally well in the two ears. This may ensure that (1) sound will be detected in at least one of the ears, notwithstanding the direction of the sound, (2) the speaker can be localized more quickly so that lip-reading cues may be used, and (3) the signal is separated from the competing noise. Computer assisted sound measurement equipment is now available for quickly matching hearing aid outputs in the two ears, as well as for determining the comparative benefits of various aid settings and earmold modifications in one ear (Fig. 6–12).

In some instances a child should be fitted monaurally rather than binaurally. Two aids should not be fitted when one ear has middle ear disease with discharge. Binaural fitting should be questioned when the unaided detection thresholds for the two ears are grossly discrepant. There are many guidelines for which ear to fit with a hearing aid if only one impaired ear is fitted.

If a child with a unilateral hearing loss is fitted, the ear with the loss is used. A contralateral routing of signals (CROS) hearing aid has also been specially designed for a child with a unilateral hearing loss (Fig. 6–13). It includes two BTE units, with an interconnecting wire. One unit includes a microphone and fits behind the impaired ear. The other unit includes the amplifier and speaker and fits behind the normal ear. Sound from the impaired ear side of the head enters the micro-

132 Facilitating Classroom Listening

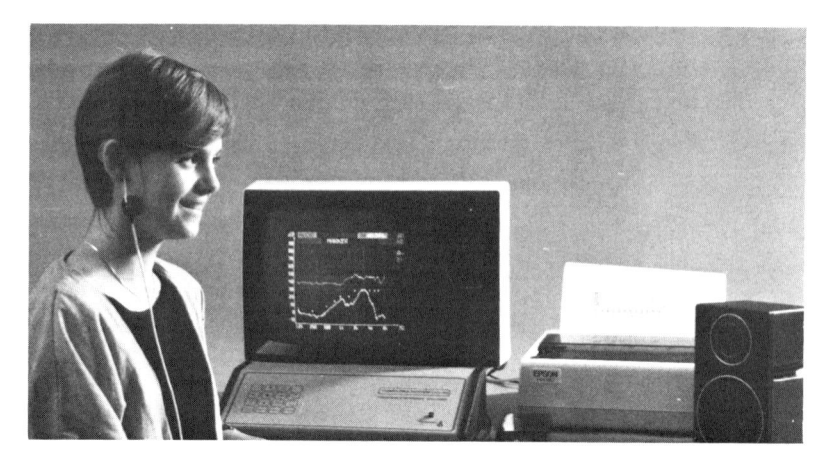

Figure 6-12. A "live" configuration and a hard copy of data for determining appropriateness of hearing aid fittings. From Rastronics advertisement. Mountainside, NJ: Rastronics. Reprinted by permission.

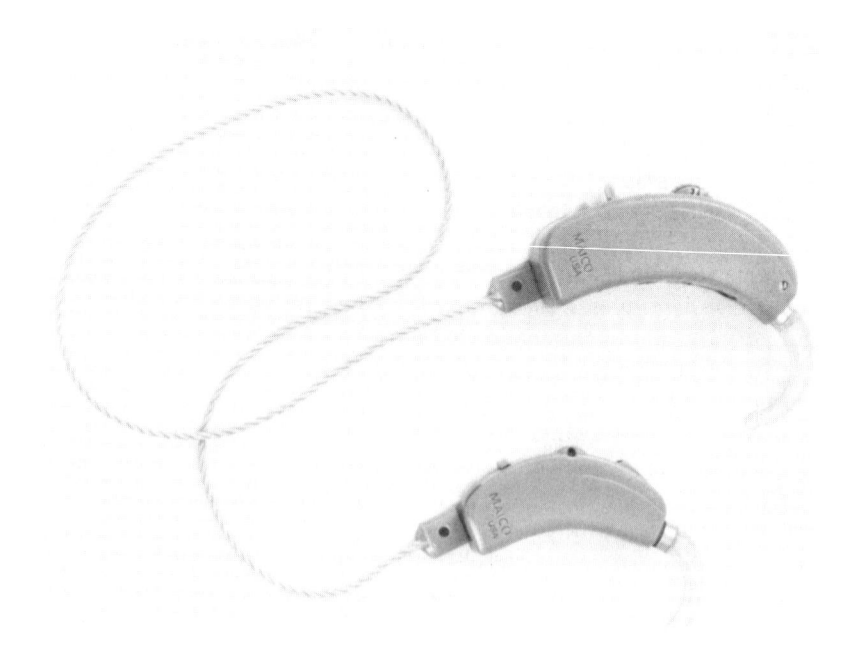

Figure 6-13. Two units and interconnecting wire of CROS aid. From Maico technical specifications of M211 hearing aid. Minneapolis: Maico Hearing Instruments. Reprinted by permission.

phone of the first unit, is electrically routed to the amplifier of the second unit, and is there transduced back into sound via the receiver. An open mold permits entry of amplified sound from the impaired ear side of the head and unamplified sound from the normal side. Only the earhook for the normal ear functions to conduct sound.

Components of a Hearing Aid

A hearing aid includes four basic components (Fig. 6-14). The first component is the microphone, which transduces incoming sound into an electrical signal. The second component is the amplifier, which increases the gain of the electrical signal but also modifies it in many other ways. The third component is the receiver, which transduces the amplified electrical signal to outgoing sound. The fourth component is the battery, which provides the electrical power for transduction, amplification, and other functions. The outgoing sound is then delivered through an earhook, tube, and earmold or shell into the ear canal.

Each hearing aid includes one or more controls. A gain (volume) control can be adjusted by the hearing aid user. Other hearing aid controls (gain, output, compression, tone or frequency) are screwdriver controls. Hearing aid switches are less commonly used. Often a BTE aid has an on-off switch or an off-microphone-telephone switch. ITE aids do not commonly have these switches. Each aid has a battery compartment, which can be opened. These and other features of BTE and ITE aids are seen in Figure 6-15.

Directional Microphone

A directional microphone can be used in a hearing aid. It allows full amplification of signals from the front, which are usually desirable signals, and simultaneously reduces amplification of signals from the rear, which often are competing unwanted signals (noise). The net

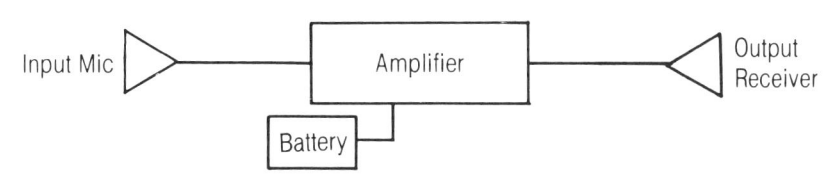

Figure 6-14. Block diagram of a hearing aid.

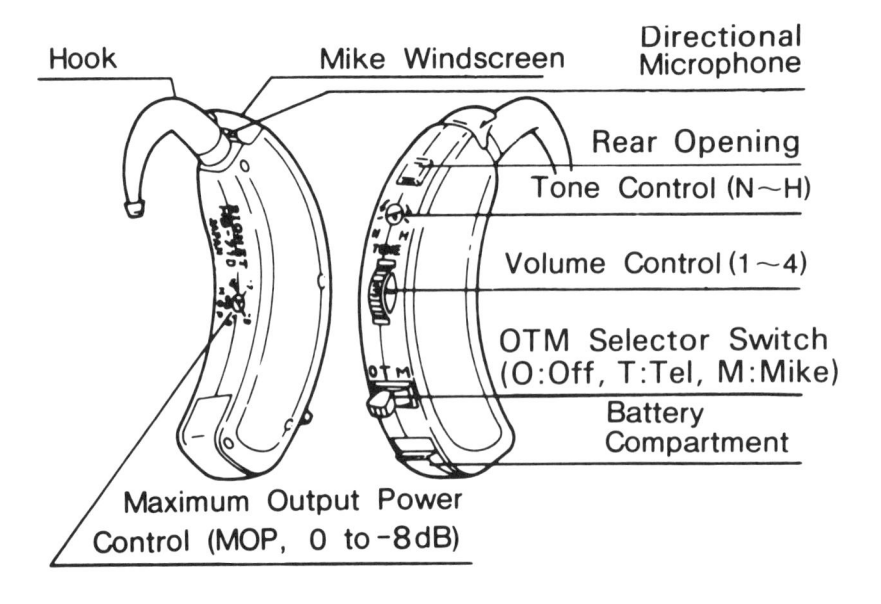

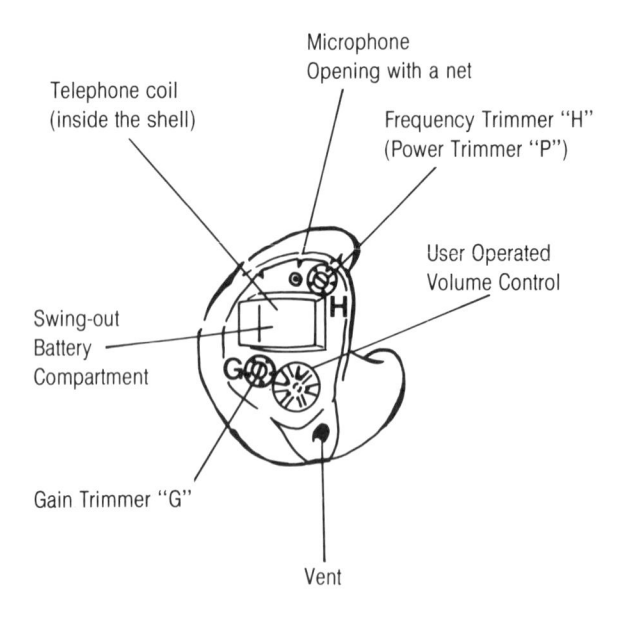

Figure 6-15. Visible controls, switches, and other features of a behind-the-ear (BTE) aid and an in-the-ear (ITE) aid. From Rion technical specifications of HB-71D and HI-03 standard ITE hearing aids. Torrance, CA: Rion Acoustics Instruments. Reprinted by permission.

result is an increase in the primary signal (message) to secondary signal (competition) ratio, or signal-to-noise (S/N) ratio, providing an opportunity for increased understanding of the message. The increase in the S/N ratio achieved with a directional microphone as compared with a standard nondirectional microphone is seen in Figure 6–16. Its use may result in an increase in speech recognition in many noisy situations. The effect is not dramatic but may be significant. The need for a directional microphone is with a BTE aid, in which the microphone faces forward. The microphone of the ITE aid faces outward.

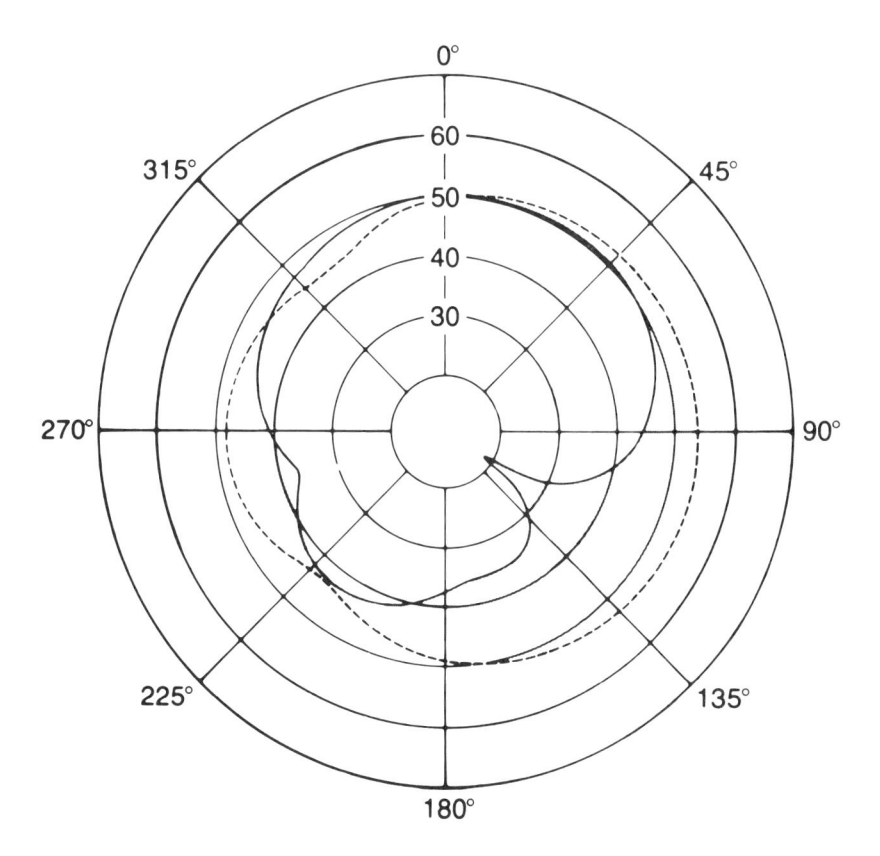

Figure 6-16. Sensitivity patterns for a directional microphone (*solid line*) and nondirectional microphone (*dotted line*). From Maico technical specifications of M211 hearing aid. Minneapolis: Maico Hearing Instruments. Reprinted by permission.

Telecoil

A telecoil can be built into either a BTE aid or an ITE aid. This allows reception of a telephone receiver signal and an FM receiver signal. Telecoil input is free from acoustic feedback and environmental noise but is not without limitations. The strength of the input depends on the number of turns in the coil, the amount of magnetic leakage from the telephone receiver, the orientation of the telecoil to the telephone receiver, and the nearness of the telecoil to the magnetic induction loop of the FM receiver.

Many newer telephones, particularly the pushbutton and trimline varieties, use components that provide too little magnetic leakage for a strong telecoil signal to be generated, unless a separate amplifier is provided. An amplifier can be built into the receiver or body of a telephone, or attached to the telephone receiver, to permit the hearing impaired child to hear better through the hearing aid telecoil or microphone, or even without a hearing aid. Figure 6-17 shows several amplification options that are commerically available.

A BTE aid is large enough to permit an off-microphone-telecoil (OMT) switch to be built into it. An OMT switch permits the user to

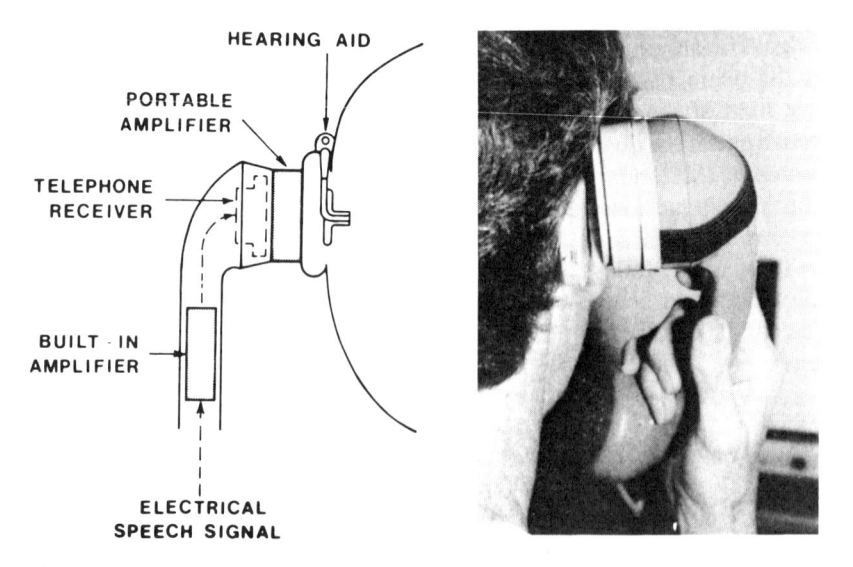

Figure 6-17. Built-in and strapped-on telephone amplifier options with behind-the-ear (BTE) hearing aids. From Erber, N. (1985). *Telephone communication and hearing impairment* (p. 22, 25). San Diego: College-Hill Press. Copyright 1985 by College-Hill Press. Reprinted by permission.

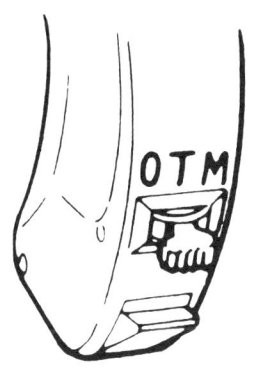

Figure 6-18. An off-microphone-telecoil (OMT) selector switch with operational instructions. From Rion technical specifications of HB-69 series hearing aids. Torrance, CA: Rion Acoustics Instruments. Reprinted by permission.

listen through either microphone input or telecoil input. In Figure 6–15, the ITE aid is shown with a telecoil but not a switch. Without a switch, a user listens to microphone input sound and simultaneously to a magnetic input signal when a telephone receiver is held up to the ear, or when a magnetic induction loop of an FM receiver is near the telecoil. Preferably, a hearing aid would enable automatic switching from microphone to telecoil input, depending on which arrangement provides the strongest and least distorted input. Switches are currently available that permit the user to choose between microphone input, telecoil input, and both in combination. Figure 6–18 explains how to use the more commonly used OMT switch, which the user manipulates.

Noise Control

Noise interference with the signal is a significant problem with a hearing aid. One major aspect of this problem is low frequency room noise that enters the microphone along with the speech signal. The ear does not respond to the very low frequency room noise. Higher low frequency room noise, however, has a masking effect upon speech. Three techniques for alleviating low frequency noise are (1) adjusting a low tone control to limit low frequency amplification, (2) increasing the diameter of a vent in an earmold or shell to drain low frequencies, and (3) using an automatic noise suppressor circuit to reduce low frequency amplification (Fig. 6–19).

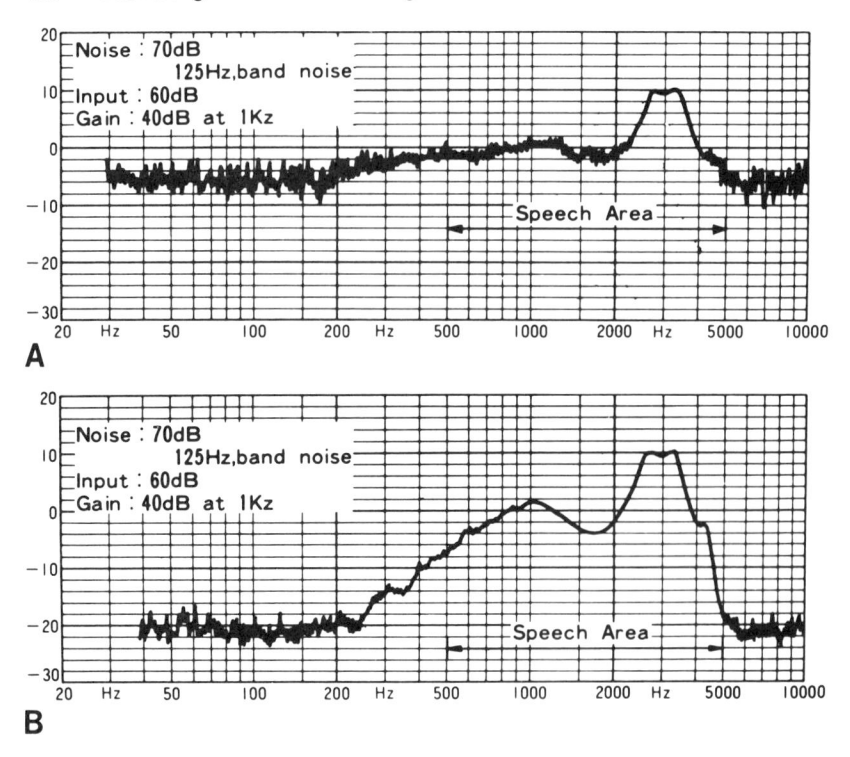

Figure 6-19. Hearing aid response with automatic noise suppression switch off (A) and on (B). From technical specifications of HB69AS hearing aid. Torrance, CA: Rion Acoustics Instruments. Reprinted by permission.

When a room is occupied by people, middle and high frequency noise also enters the microphone of a hearing aid. Currently, this noise cannot be separated from the signal. Separation may be achieved, at least to some extent, when digital hearing aids become commercially available. A digital hearing aid is a computer-based system that replaces statndard electronic components. With computer software and tiny chips of exceedingly complex circuitry, a very advanced program for digitally manipulating the signal is possible. The hearing aid response will conform more exactly to the individualized hearing needs of each hearing aid user.

Noise also exists when incoming sound is compressed in a hearing aid. Momentary sound blackouts occur when there are sudden loud sounds. Pumping sounds are also characteristic of compression circuits. A new and more complex type of compression circuit called adaptive compression, appropriately regulates the time a hearing aid is in

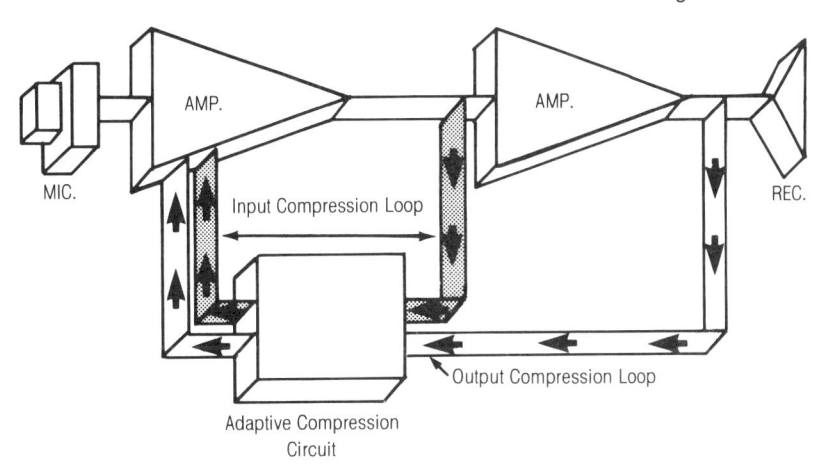

Figure 6-20. A block diagram of an adaptive compression hearing aid. From advertisement on Telex 363C aid. Minneapolis: Telex Communication. Reprinted by permission.

compression, eliminating the sound blackouts and pumping sounds. This is demonstrated on a tape recording called "Hearing is Believing," available from Telex Hearing Aids. Adaptive compression is available for BTE or ITE aids (Fig. 6–20).

HEARING AND MANAGEMENT PROGRAMS

The audiologist is responsible for determining the candidacy of a child for hearing aids; selecting the most appropriate available aids; securing the most appropriate BTE earmolds or ITE shells; fitting and adjusting the aids and molds; counseling and training parents, teachers, and the child on the use of this equipment; and managing these devices. Hearing aids are built to last, but they are complicated and vulnerable to wear and tear. At one moment an aid may work well, and the next moment or shortly thereafter, it may not. Children are particularly hard on hearing aids because they are carefree and active. Consequently, children tend to have hearing aids that do not work optimally, unless a hearing aid management program is operational. An informed, systematic, and sustained hearing aid management program is needed in the schools.

A hearing aid management program is a part of the overall IEP written and implemented for a hearing handicapped child. The management program requires the cooperation of the child, the parents, the teachers, the principal, the audiologist who dispenses and services hearing aids, the hearing aid manufacturer, and the educational audiologist or speech-language pathologist. Prior to returning an aid to a manufacturer for servicing, visual and listening checks on the aid need to be performed at school or at home, and local servicing needs to be performed. It is preferable that the dispensing audiologist have a test box for evaluating the physical characteristics of a hearing aid and a battery current drain meter. The dispensing audiologist should also have basic hearing aid evaluation and maintenance equipment.

Hearing aid characteristics measured with the test box include maximum power output, gain, frequency response, distortion, compression, internal noise, and telecoil strength. When a hearing aid is first purchased, its physical characteristics should be determined by the audiologist before being fitted on a child. When children are young or particularly careless with their aids, test box checks should be conducted monthly or whenever a hearing aid problem is uncovered through a visual or listening check. When children are older or are careful with their aids, test box checks should be performed annually. When an aid has been sent to the service department of the hearing aid company and returned, the performance characteristics should be checked. In a recent study of hearing aids after repair, an audiologist found that most aids did not approximate original manufacturer's specifications for physical characteristics, and 15 percent had to be returned to the factory for further repair. Figure 6–21 shows a portable test box and a more sophisticated clinical test box, with printers. In the service department of a hearing aid factory, advanced analysis equipment is systematically used.

The dispensing audiologist who does not have a test box can perform a quick but detailed listening check to identify hearing aid problems. Specific listening check procedures have been developed for estimating hearing aid function: gain, power output, frequency response, S/N ratio, and distortion. These checks are important, because often when an aid is sent back to the factory, no specific technical problem is identified. In the management of hearing aids, the dispensing audiologist also performs simple upkeep of aids and makes ear impressions for replacement of BTE earmolds and ITE shells. This service work may be included as a part of the purchase price of the aid or may be done at relatively low cost afterwards. Local servicing should be done very promptly so the aid can be kept on the the child.

Hearing aid manufacturers provide 1 to 3 year warranties on hearing aids purchased. They also provide quick turnaround time on service of hearing aids. Aids mailed to the factory are often returned within a week. If a child has binaural aids, only one aid should be sent to the factory at a time. If a child has only one aid, the dispensing audiologist may

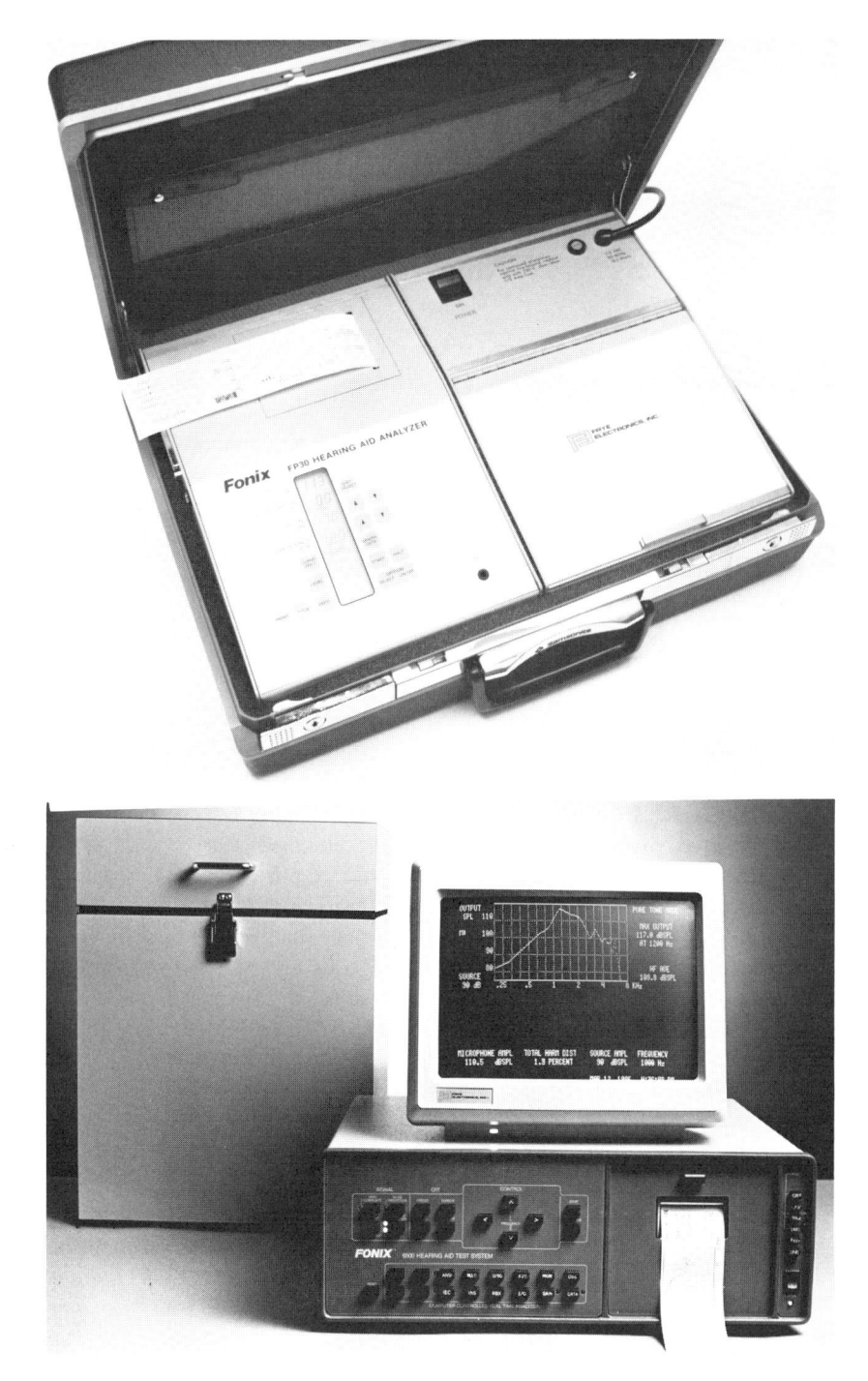

Figure 6-21. Portable and clinical test box systems with chambers, analyzers, and printers. From technical specifications on FONIX FP 30 and FONIX 6500 hearing aid test systems. Tigard, OR: Frye Electronics. Reprinted by permission.

temporarily lend an aid. The earmold of the original hearing aid, if a BTE aid, can be connected to the loaner aid. The shell of a modular ITE aid can also be connected to a loaner aid. The shell of a custom ITE aid cannot be separated from the aid and replaced with another shell.

Daily Checking and Servicing

Daily visual checks and listening checks of students' hearing aids should be conducted by parents, classroom teachers, or the students themselves. A visual check is inspecting each externally visible part of an aid for problems. A listening check is listening to the sound output of the hearing aid for problems, while manipulating the sound input and controls of the aid. Some problems can be seen, but more can be heard. Initially, a person needs to see and listen to the aid while it is functioning properly to have a basis for finding problems. A visual check of an aid takes only a minute. A complete listening check takes longer. A parent, teacher, or older student needs to spend a few minutes at the beginning of a school day in checking and servicing an aid. At the end of the day, the voltage of the battery of an aid needs to be checked also. If the aid is dirty, it should be cleaned. If another problem is discovered, that problem should be quickly remedied.

Checking and servicing a hearing aid requires the use of simple devices and inexpensive materials, and following specific procedures. Figure 6–22 shows cleaning and replacement materials that were originally selected in a school district for BTE aids but can be used for ITE aids as well.

Additional cleaning materials are included in an ITE kit (Fig. 6–23). The ITE cleaner kit includes a wave remover wire wire loop, a pick for removing wax from hard to reach areas or for bending small parts, and a minibrush for removing debris in or around a microphone opening. Cetylcide spray is also included. It should be wiped dry with a tissue.

Most hearing aid problems are mechanical rather than electronic: for instance, faulty volume controls and switches, broken wires, defective solder connections, wax in the earmold or receiver outlet, intermittent battery contacts, and moisture. Modern electronic components such as transducers, resistors, capacitors, and integrated circuits, are extremely reliable and troublefree. A number of specific problems and remedies that should be known to teachers. parents, and the hearing impaired will now be discussed: moisture, batteries, causes of dead aids, squeal, and user complaints about sound.

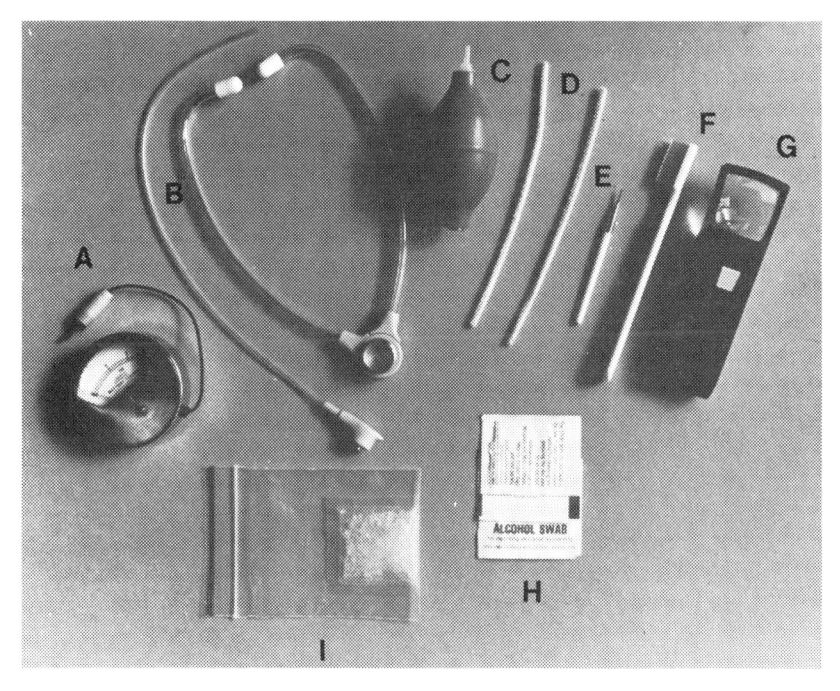

Figure 6-22. Hearing aid maintenance kit. (A) battery tester. (B) hearing aid stethoscope and adaptor. (C) forced-air earmold cleaner. (D) pipe cleaners. (E) small, soft brush. (F) child-size toothrbrush. (G) lighted magnifying glass. (H) individual packets of alcohol saturated swabs. (I) packets of silica gel and a lock-top plastic bag. From Musket, C. (1981). Maintenance of personal hearing aids. In R. Roeser and M. Downs (Eds.), *Auditory disorders in school children* (p. 239). New York: Thieme-Stratton. Copyright 1981 by Thieme-Stratton.

Moisture

Moisture is the most common cause of hearing aid failure. If moisture can penetrate a hearing aid, it can affect both mechanical and electronic functions. Sweaty physical activity or even wet and humid weather conditions are sources of damaging moisture and corrosive salt.

There are different approaches to protecting an aid from moisture (Fig. 6–24). A new product, Moisture Guard, can be wrapped daily around the aid. Another new product, Super Dri-Aid, includes pellets that absorb moisture overnight from a hearing aid. The aid is placed on a foam pad in a sealed jar containing the pellets. One hearing aid is built to be moisture-proof. Neophrene seals are used to protect the interior parts.

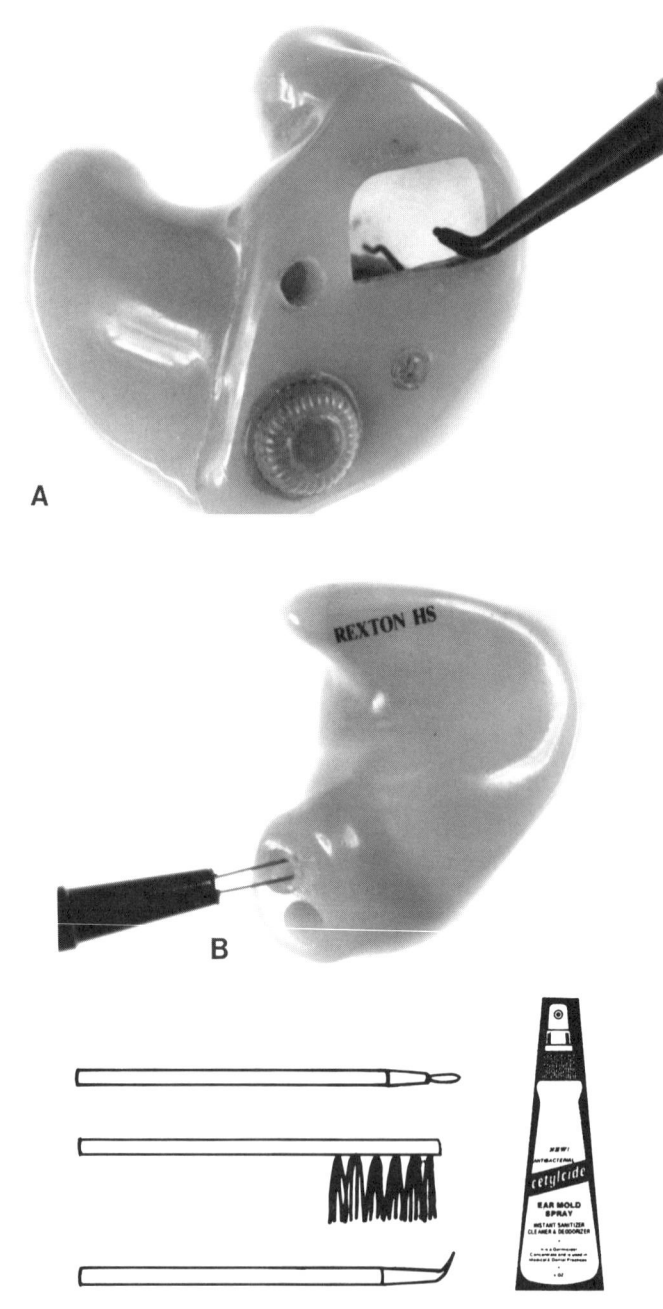

Figure 6-23. (A) Using a toothpick to bend battery contacts of an in-the-ear (ITE) aide back into place. (B) Using a wax removal tool to remove ear wax from the receiver tube of an ITE aid. From Agnew, J. (1985). In-office analysis of malfunctioning ITE aids. *Hearing instruments, 36,* 20. Reprinted by permission. (C) An ITE cleaner kit. Kit includes one wax remover, one all-purpose pick, and one mini-brush. From Hal-Hen literature. Long Island, NY: Hal-Hen Company. Reprinted by permission.

Figure 6-24. See page 146 for legend.

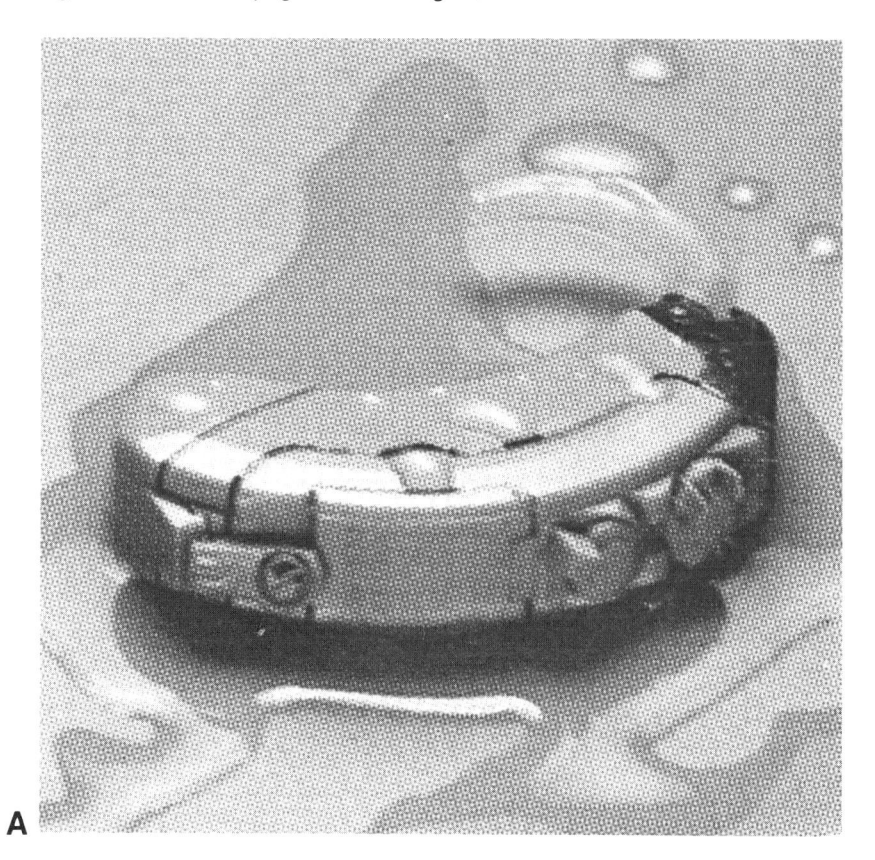

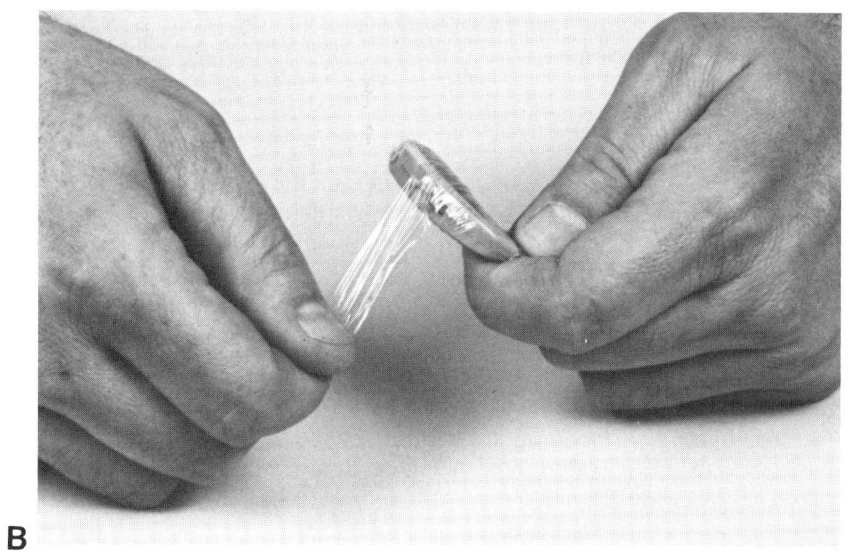

A

B

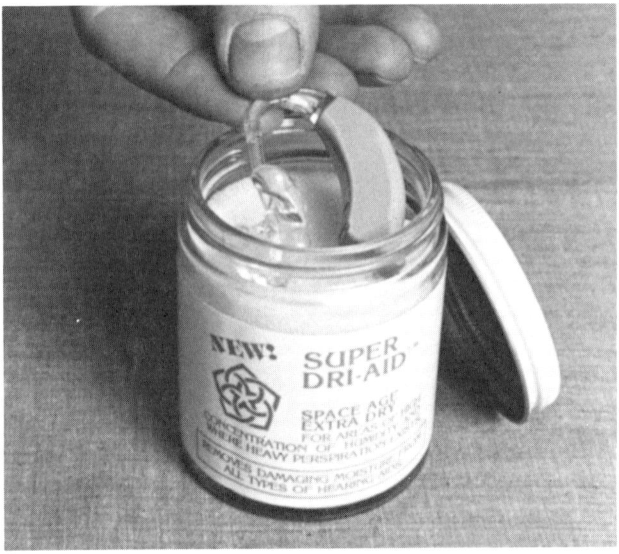

C

Figure 6-24. (A) A moisture-proof hearing aid. From flyer on Rion HB-35 hearing aid. Torrance, CA: Rion Acoustic Instruments. Reprinted by permission. (B) Moisture Guard. (C) Placing an aid inside a jar that has Super-Dri-Aid pellets. From Hal-Hen literature. Long Island, NY: Hal-Hen Company. Reprinted by permission.

An airtight battery compartment has been built. The trimmer controls are water resistant and dust proof. A water inhibiting fabric is included in the microphone screen.

Batteries

The battery that powers the hearing aid is a major service problem. A battery has a limited life. It may be defective before it is ever inserted in the aid. It can become corroded. If a battery is not inserted in a battery compartment carefully, the battery contacts can become disaligned. A detached battery and a dead hearing aid are the result.

Battery life ordinarily depends on the gain of the hearing aid or type of battery. A low gain instrument will not drain as much current per hour as a high gain instrument. A zinc air battery will last longer than a mercury battery. A low gain aid with the most efficient zinc air battery may last more than 1000 hours. A high gain aid with a mercury battery may last no longer than 70 hours. Zinc air batteries are covered with a seal. As soon as the seal is detached, the battery very slowly begins to

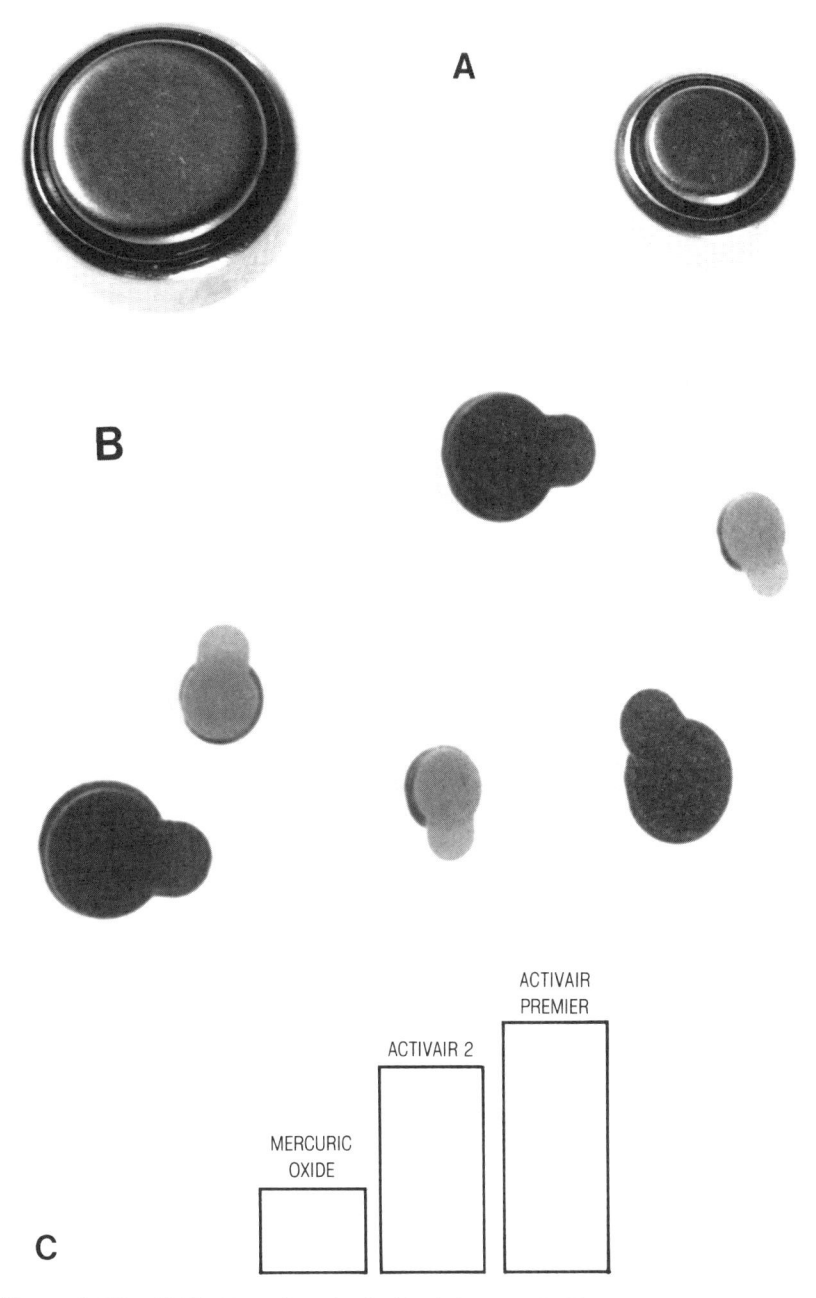

Figure 6-25. (A) Battery sizes for behind-the-ear (BTE) and in-the-ear (ITE) hearing aids. (B) Sealed zinc air batteries. (C) Comparative battery life. From Activar zinc air battery advertisement. Eagen, MN: Acitvar Division, Duracell. Reprinted by permission.

lose capacity. Figure 6-25 shows various batteries, the seals on zinc air batteries, and comparative life of mercury and zinc air batteries.

Battery life will be shorter than it should be if the battery is defective or the gain is set too high. The user may set the gain higher than it needs to be, to compensate for a plugged receiver tube or plugged earmold bore. An audiologist uses a special meter to measure the drain of current from a battery placed in the hearing aid. The audiologist can compute the number of hours the battery is going to last and compare that with the manufacturer's battery life specifications.

Visual inspection and service begins with the battery. Open the battery compartment and check for corrosion. If a battery is heavily corroded, the battery should be discarded. Be sure to keep discarded batteries in a safe place away from little children. Any corrosion on battery contacts should be wiped clean with a soft cloth, an alcohol swab, or a pencil eraser.

Check also to be sure that an appropriate size battery is used. Ordinarily a size 675 battery is used with a BTE aid and a size 13 with a standard ITE aid. Check also that the battery is installed properly, with the + side of the battery aligned with the + marking stamped or engraved in the battery compartment.

Use a battery tester to check the voltage of the battery, preferably after it has been used all day. The battery should be replaced if the voltage reading is 0.2 to 0.3 volts below the manufacturer's battery specification, which is usually about 1.35 volts.

In testing a battery, place the negative terminal of the battery tester to the negative side of the battery. Likewise, place the positive terminal of the battery tester to the positive side of the battery. The needle of the battery tester will deflect from its 0 position to the right and indicate the battery foltage. Digital battery testers will indicate battery voltage directly.

Dead Aids

A dead battery is just one of the causes of a dead hearing aid. Table 6-1 lists six causes of dead aids and gives local remedies. Two causes relate to batteries, three to sound stoppage, and one to disconnection of parts. The teacher, parent, or user can remedy the simpler problems and leave the more difficult problems to the audiologist. Remedies for many other causes of dead batteries require servicing from the manufacturers.

After cerumen or foreign material has been removed from a hearing aid or earmold, remaining debris should be cleaned out as well as possible. The earmold of a BTE aid can be detached from a tubing, a pipe cleaner pushed through the sound bore, and the earmold washed with warm water and mild soap and dried afterwards with a forced-air

Table 6-1. Causes and Local Remedies for Dead ITE and BTE Aids

Cause	Remedy
Dead battery	Use a battery tester to find a fresh aid from the battery stock
Battery contacts or battery dirty	Clean with pencil eraser or with cotton-tipped applicator, sparingly dipped in isopropyl alcohol
Cerumen plugging an ITE receiver tube or a BTE earmold sound bore	Carefully use a wax removal tool to remove cerumen; do not puncture or tear tube or bore
Debris in microphone port of BTE or ITE aid or in receiver port of ITE aid	Carefully remove with tweezers; be careful not to push further into port
Earmold tubing or earhook has come loose	Replace with new tubing or earhook

From Agnew, J. (1985). In-office analysis of malfunctioning ITE aids. *Hearing Instruments, 36,* 22. Adapted by permission.

earmold cleaner. Cetylide spray can also be used to clean and deodorize earmolds and tubing. The forced air cleaner can also be used to dry out tubing. If the tubing is hardened, cracked, or otherwise defective, it can be replaced by the audiologist. If an earhook needs to be replaced, this can also be done by the audiologist.

Squeal

A listening check of a hearing aid includes checking for acoustic feedback. This is continual leakage of amplified sound back into the microphone of a hearing aid. The hearing aid in turn amplifies or resonates, causing an extraneous squeal, howl, or whistling sound. Acoustic feedback causes a problem to both the hearing aid user and other people who are annoyed by the sound. Steps the audiologist takes in correcting acoustic feedback in a BTE aid are detailed here. The teacher should be aware of the steps but need not be directly involved.

> The first step in correcting a problem relating to feedback is to assess the source of the acoustic leak. The acoustic leak may occur between the earmold and the ear canal from a poorly fitted earmold. The acoustic leak may also result from a vent which is too large . . . from loose or broken earmold tubing, from a loose or broken earhook, or from loose or disconnected tubing between the receiver and the nozzle. The audiologist must simply work from the earmold backward, closing off the earmold, tubing, and earhook, until the feedback is eliminated. For example, if the feedback is eliminated when the audiologist closes off the sound bore vent of the earmold, the feedback can be assumed to be the result of a poorly fitting earmold or a vent

which is too large. If the feedback is still present when the sound bore and vent are occluded, then the source of the feedback must necessarily be between the earmold and the hearing aid. The next step is to remove the tubing from the earhook, occlude the end of the earhook, and again check for feedback. If feedback is not present with the earhook occluded, the source of the feedback is the tubing. If feedback is still present, the source of the feedback is between the earhook and the hearing aid. The next step is to remove the earhook and occlude the receiver nozzle. If the feedback is thereby eliminated, the source of the feedback is the earhook. If the feedback is not eliminated, the source of the feedback is internal and the hearing aid should be sent to the manufacturer for repair. Once the source of the feedback is determined, the audiologist can take steps to correct the problem. It may be necessary to occlude the earmold vent, build up the earmold, or obtain a new and tighter fitting one. It may be necessary to replace the tubing and/or the earhook if these are the source of the problem. (Viehweg, 1986, p. 126)

The process of finding the source of acoustic feedback in an ITE aid is similar. With either the BTE or the ITE aid, the new silicone impression material reduces feedback from a poorly fitting mold or shell. If feedback is due to a vent that is too large, vent plugs can be inserted, a small piece of acoustic foam can be placed in the vent, a tone trimmer adjusted, or the gain of the aid reduced. BTE earmolds or ITE shells for children with severe and profound bilateral loss do not have vents. These children have to learn to get along with a stuffy, full feeling in their ear canals when using an earmold or shell.

Listening Stethoscope

A listening check mainly involves use of a stethoscope, adapter, and connecting tube. As seen in Figure 6–26, a nozzle on one end of the connecting tube is slipped over the canal portion of a BTE earmold or ITE shell. The other end of the connecting tube is atached to the stethoscope adapter. The ear pieces of the stethoscope are inserted in the ears of the listener. The outside of the mold or shell may be sanitized with cetylcide spray.

In checking the aid, with a stethoscope, initially the aid should be turned on. If the aid has a telephone-microphone switch, it should be in the microphone position. Begin with the volume control turned down. Do not say anything, but listen to the internal noise of the hearing aid circuit. A low level, smooth hissing sound is normally heard. If a high level hiss, or sputtering, popping, crackling or other random and objectionable noise is heard, the aid should be returned to the factory for internal repairs.

Next, say words like *test* and *five* repeatedly, while listening to the aid and varying the volume control wheel. By turning the volume control up and down, dead spots in rotation or a noisy volume control ele-

A

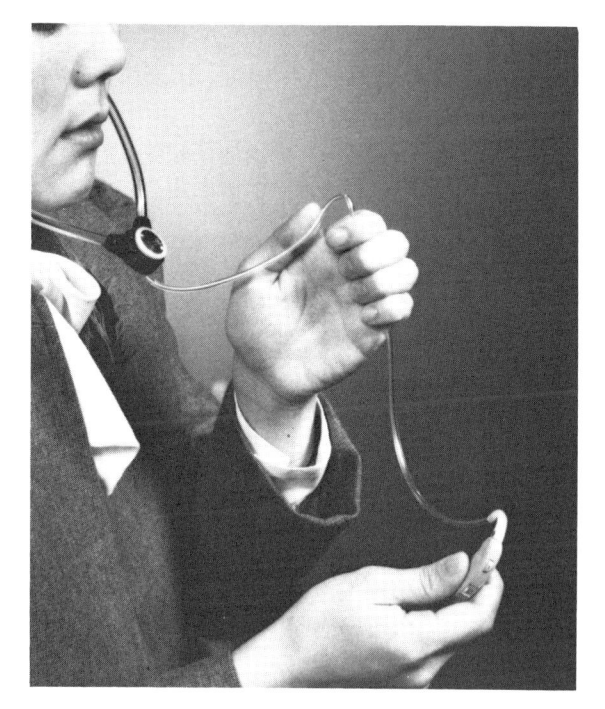

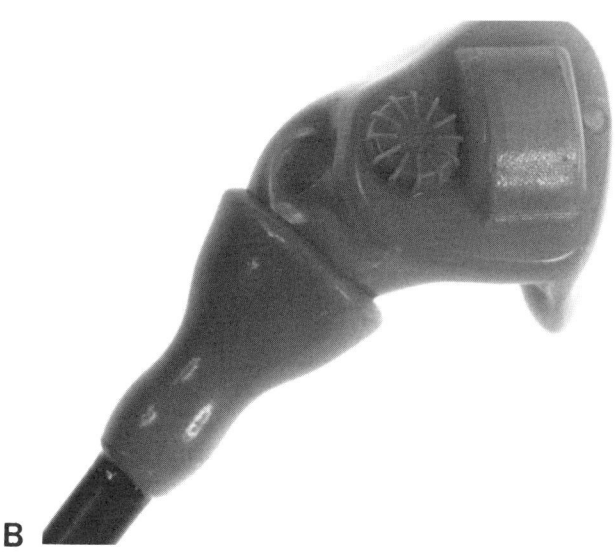

B

Figure 6-26. (A) Stethoscope attached to behind-the-ear (BTE) aid. From Duhamel, G., and Yoshioka, P. (1985). Subjective listening techniques for assessing hearing aid function. *Hearing Instruments, 36,* 20. Reprinted by permission. (B) Stethoscope attached to ITE aid. From Agnew, J. (1985). In-office analysis of malfunctioning ITE aids. *Hearing Instruments, 36,* 20. Reprinted by permission.

ment can be identified. A liquid called "No Noise" sprayed on this element may cure the problem.

If distortion or an improper frequency response exists in the aid, it can be identified by listening to the words *test* and *five* because their sounds approximate the intensities and frequencies of overall speech. Short bursts of monotone whistle also help in recognizing distortion.

Various hearing aid problems may be identified from corresponding sounds heard in the stethoscope check. Distorted sound may mean that moisture or debris is on the diaphragm of the microphone or receiver, that a diaphragm is cracked, or that a volume control is turned up too high, clipping off the peaks of sounds. Excessive hissing may mean that too much internal noise is being generated by the microphone of the aid. Buzzing may mean that a battery is weak or an electronic circuit defective.

Hearing aid users may complain that they hear various strange sounds when their aids are not adjusted properly. A list of user complaints about sound of ITE aids, causes, and remedies is shown in Table 6–2. A similar list of complaints, causes, and remedies could be generated for BTE aids. The remedies should be provided by the audiologist who fitted the aid.

The next step in the stethoscope check is to rotate the volume control to the point where it is used by the hearing aid user. Let another person say the sounds "oo, ah, ee, sh, and s" from 3 feet away, or average conversational distance. Optionally, play back a tape recording of these sounds at this distance. These sounds have been discussed as the five test sound test in Chapter 4. Each should be detected if the frequency response of the hearing aid extends from 500 to 4000 Hz.

SUMMARY

A hearing aid may be beneficial for nearly all children with a permanent or long standing bilateral hearing loss, and similarly for many children with unilateral hearing loss. Both BTE and ITE aids have potential benefits for students in school. An aid can manipulate incoming sound in many ways to compensate for various degrees and configurations of hearing loss. These potential benefits for school children, however, will not be reached unless a systematic hearing aid management program is implemented. The hearing aid manufacturer, the dispensing audiologist, parents, teachers, and the hearing aid user have important roles in a management program. Daily checking and servicing of aids in integral to management success.

Table 6-2. User Complaints About Sounds of ITE Aids

Complaint	Cause	Remedy
Muffled, hollow, "in a barrel," booming	Too many low frequencies	Recheck audiogram and aid response curve and test the aid in a test box; if they appear correct, try adjusting the low frequency control, if there is one, and/or increase the vent size to remove some of the low frequencies
Tinny, shrill, or high pitched	Too many high frequencies	Recheck audiogram and original fitting specifications and test hearing aid; if these appear correct, try adding more low frequencies by adjusting the low frequency control or by decreasing the vent size with vent plugs
	Borderline feedback	Check causes of feedback
	User not used to high frequencies	User education; add low frequencies with response control until user is used to the aid; alternatively, decrease vent size
Stuffy feeling, fullness in ear	Lack of venting	If aid has no vent, add one; increase existing vent size; check to see if vent is plugged
Insufficient volume, even though aid meets factory specifications	Incorrect frequency response	Recheck audiogram and original response specification
	Incorrect gain specification	Recheck audiogram and original gain specification
Wind noise	Blowing wind	Try a small piece of foam or lamb's wool in the microphone port, being careful not to push it in too far

From Agnew, J. (1985). In-office analysis of malfunctioning ITE aids. *Hearing Instruments, 36,* 28. Reprinted by permission.

FURTHER READINGS

Michael Pollack's book entitled *Amplification for the Hearing Impaired* (Grune & Stratton, New York, 1980) is a comprehensive reference on hearing aids. The *Vanderbilt Hearing Aid Report* (Upper Darby, PA, 1982), edited by Gerald Studebaker and Frederick Bess, describes more recent advances in hearing aid technology. Steven

Viehweg's chapter on hearing aids in the book *Educational Audiology for the Hard of Hearing Child* (Grune & Stratton, Orlando, FL, 1986), edited by Frederick Berg, James Blair, Steven Viehweg, and Ann Wilson-Vlotman, provides a concise treatise on hearing aids for school children. Maintenance of personal hearing aids in the schools is covered well by Caroline Muskett in a chapter of the book *Auditory Disorders in School Children* (Thieme-Stratton, New York, 1981), edited by Ross Roeser and Marion Downs.

Chapter 7

FM Equipment

CASE STUDY

MH is a 10 year old girl in the fourth grade. She has a sensorineural bilateral hearing loss. Her audiograms reveal average detection thresholds of 30 dB in the left ear and 35 dB in the right ear. MH appears to have had hearing impairment from birth. An audiologist diagnosed her loss when she was 4 years old. At that time she was referred for hearing testing because her verbal development and communication were depressed. The audiologist, and an otologist who also tested MH, recommended binaural hearing aids. However, MH's parents would not support her wearing aids because aids would make her "look funny." Her parents did agree to buy a hearing aid that could be used for "communication therapy." MH also used the aid for communication practice at home.

MH then attended preschool. When she was 6, her parents enrolled her in kindergarten. MH was bright but "just got by" in school. MH could not keep up with her peers in learning new words. She just did not hear enough of what was going on around her.

MH has learned to read orally and comprehends first and second grade reading material. She is having difficulty comprehending third and fourth grade reading material. A speech-language pathologist now gives her private communication training at home. MH is still using her hearing aid only for training.

The district where MH attends school has a speech-language pathologist, who could have been assigned to help her. MH's parents, however, have refused to allow her to receive special help in school. They have said they did not want MH to be taken out of her class. The school principal has now informed MH's parents that MH may have to be held back a year in school.

MH's parents are now reconsidering what is best for her. They have admitted that a hearing aid would have helped MH but that group acceptance was more important. Perhaps now would be a good time to have MH wear aids. The speech-language pathologist explained to them that FM equipment would also help MH. It would enable her to understand teachers from across the room, whereas hearing aids would let her understand only at conversational distances.

MH's parents recently saw a classroom demonstration of sound field FM equipment. The teacher wore a microphone, and her voice was transmitted and heard through loudspeakers. All the students in class could hear her, even a hearing aid user who was across the room from the teacher. They all liked the FM equipment. The teacher was also happy because she did not have to raise her voice to be heard. Another good thing about FM was that it made the classroom quieter. Soft music was played over the FM to reward the students for being quiet. The students took turns reading in front of the class using the FM microphone. Each student could be heard clearly by his or her classmates, which enhanced attention. The principal and other teachers at the school saw the demonstration and said that every classroom should be equipped with FM.

Afterwards, MH's parents saw a classroom demonstration of personal FM equipment. A teacher again wore a microphone, but her voice was transmitted to just one student, who was using an FM receiver. This student was a hearing impaired boy and was wearing two hearing aids. He went to different places in the classroom and was always able to repeat back what the teacher said. This boy had a more severe hearing loss than MH but was doing well in school. He had used hearing aids for many years. With his aids, he could repeat what the teacher said from a close distance but not from across the room, unless he was looking at the teacher.

MH's parents now realize that they have let her down because of their misconceptions. They have decided to get her new hearing aids and either personal or sound field FM equipment.

BASIC CONSIDERATIONS

Introduction to FM Equipment

During the last 20 years FM equipment has been increasingly used with hearing impaired children in schools. Initially, it was used in place of hearing aids. More recently, FM equipment has been used together with hearing aids. Still more recently, FM equipment has been used with entire classes of students, including normally hearing youngsters.

FM is an acronym for frequency modulation. This is a term applied to radio transmission of signals. A speech or other sound signal, after being changed into an electrical signal, is superimposed on a radio signal, which is transmitted. This superimposition is referred to as modulating the radio signal. The amplitude of the radio signal can be modulated (AM) or the frequency of the radio signal can be modulated (FM). A sound transmitter sends out AM or FM radio waves, and a radio receiver picks them up and delivers them to listeners.

Figure 7-1 shows (1) an audio frequency signal, which is a low frequency signal like speech, (2) a radio frequency signal or carrier wave, which has a much higher frequency, (3) amplitude modulation of the carrier wave, and (4) frequency modulation of the carrier wave. An FM signal is preferred to an AM signal because it has better quality and is less subject to static interference.

Millions of "radios" owned by people receive both AM and FM waves. AM stations broadcast on frequencies between 535,000 and 1,605,000 Hz. The FM broadcast band extends from 88 million to 108 million Hz. A special 72,000,000 to 78,000,000 Hz band has been used for transmitting signals for the specialized FM equipment discussed in this chapter.

Radio transmission of sound has the effect of bringing the speaker to the listener. The effect is dramatic when persons listen through loudspeakers, and is even more dramatic when they listen through ear-

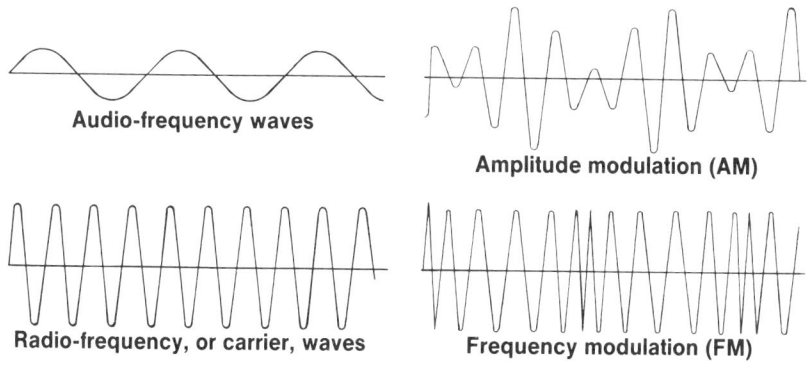

Figure 7-1. Audio and radio frequency signals separated and combined into AM and FM waves.

phones. When specialized FM equipment is used in a classroom, the teacher's voice is loud and speech is nonreverberant, especially when a listener has an earphone or a hearing aid. From across a classroom, the S/N with a loudspeaker may be 10+ dB, and with an earphone or hearing aid, 25+ dB.

These two radio options can be referred to as personal and sound field FM. When the listener uses an earphone or a hearing aid, listening is personal. When listeners hear through loudspeakers, sound is coming from the near "field."

Basically, a specialized FM system includes a microphone and transmitter, which a teacher wears, and a radio receiver. With personal FM, the listener wears the radio receiver and uses an earphone, or more frequently a personal hearing aid. With sound field FM, a common radio receiver, an amplifier, and one or more loudspeakers are used. Both personal FM and sound field FM components can be used in a classroom at the same time. Figure 7–2 shows the components of a combined personal and sound field FM arrangement.

Persons using FM transmitters can broadcast their voices from any location up to 200 feet away. Any other sound source, such as a radio or tape recorder, can also be broadcast. The radio receiver is tuned to the broadcast channel of the radio transmitter. FM listening systems can be used in different classrooms, with each system broadcasting a different radio frequency.

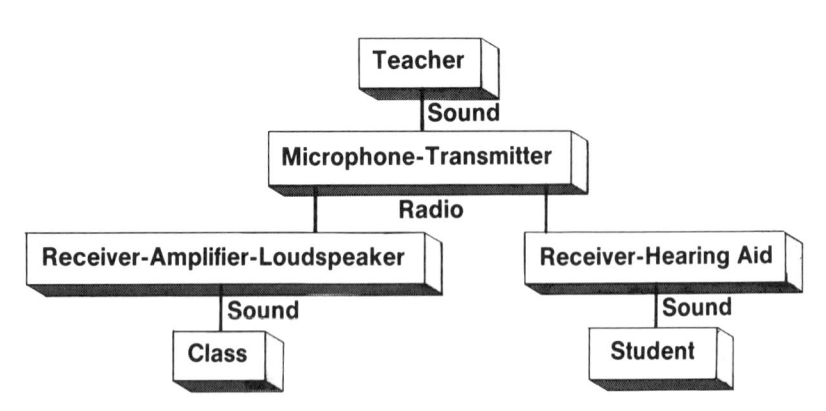

Figure 7–2. Block diagram of a classroom FM listening system including a teacher, a microphone-transmitter, personal reception equipment for a hearing aid user, and sound field reception equipment for an entire class.

Candidates for Sound Field FM

An entire regular class benefits when sound field FM equipment is installed in a classroom. The teacher can be in any location within the classroom, facing toward or away from students, and be heard consistently well. A student can also use the FM transmitter and be heard well. Sound from a tape recorder or other audiovisual device can be plugged into the system and broadcast. The gain of the amplifier can be adjusted for soft or loud sound input. The system operates best when students hear the broadcast signal no louder than 75 dB.

Often classroom noise averages 60 dBA. Without FM equipment, the teacher's voice may vary from 65 to 55 dB from the front to the back of the classroom. With FM, the teacher's voice may vary from 65 to 75 dB. The teacher's voice is clearer to students because more sounds of speech are detected. Hearing impaired students are especially benefited, including hearing aid users. A 10 dB gain makes sound ten times more intense!

A great many students in school have minimal hearing losses. School classrooms are also typically noisy and reverberant. Students are also usually seated 6 to 20 feet from a teacher. Under less than satisfactory acoustical conditions, students with minimal hearing impairment benefit greatly from sound field FM equipment. When classroom acoustics are adequate, however, these same students may do as well by turning up the gain of hearing aids. Unfortunately, adequate classroom acoustics are rare.

Most students in the regular schools who currently wear hearing aids have moderate and severe bilateral hearing losses. Their unaided detection thresholds vary from 40 to 90 dB. Their aided detection thresholds correspondingly vary from 20 to 45 dB. With the 10 dB S/N benefit provided by sound field FM equipment, hearing aid users detect a correspondingly higher percentage of speech sounds, increasing their speech recognition.

When children in school recognize speech better, they can learn more. Figure 7-3 shows academic achievement scores of minimally hearing impaired students in grades 4, 5, and 6. One group used sound field FM equipment. Another group received resource room instruction. A third group received no intervention. This study is summarized here:

> Wabash and Ohio Valley Special Education District, located in southern Illinois, conducted a three year, longitudinal study of students possessing minimal hearing loss and academic achievement deficits. The data indicate (1) 32% of the students in regular classrooms of the 4th, 5th, and 6th grades were found to have minimal hearing loss; (2) 75% of these 6th grade minimal hearing loss students had an academic deficit in one or more of the

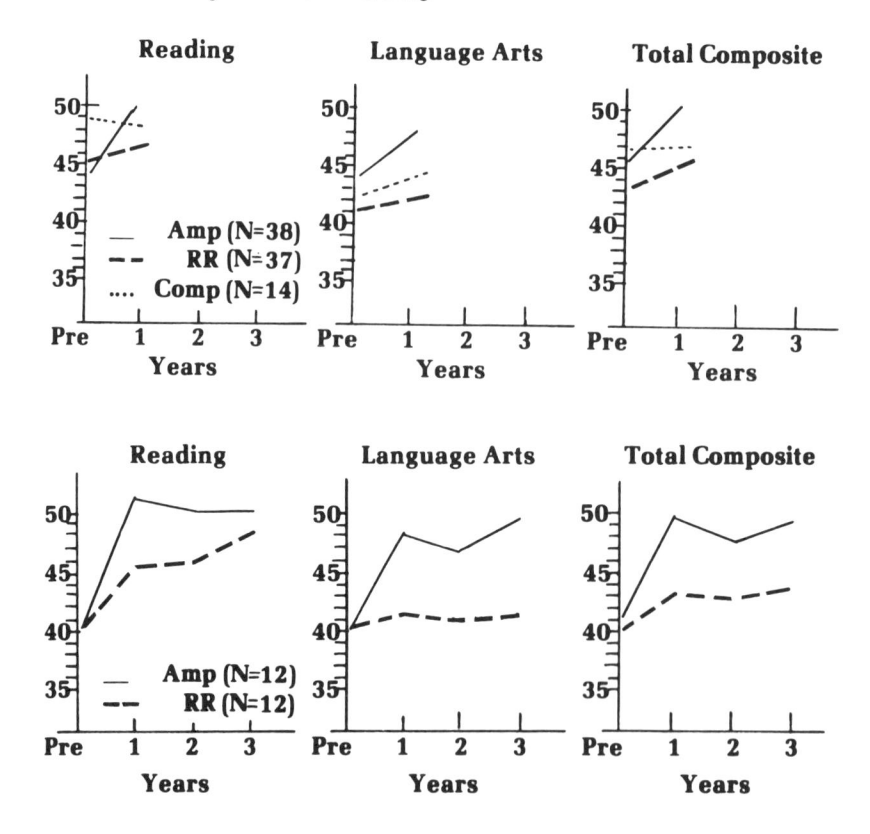

Figure 7-3. Academic achievement scores of minimally hard of hearing students before and after 1 year of treatment (A) and 3 years of treatment (B). Amp = amplified treatment, RR = resource room treatment, Comp. = comparison group with no intervention. From Sarff, L., Ray, H., and Bagwell, C. (1981). Why not amplification in every classroom? *The Hearing Aid Journal,* **34** (12): 44. Copyright 1982 by the Laux Company. Reprinted by permission.

"basic" academic skill areas of reading, language arts, or math (approximately 25% of all sixth grade students); and (3) teacher-voice amplification in the regular classroom resulted in a significant improvement in academic achievement test scores of the minimal hearing loss students. These gains were achieved within the mainstream of education at a faster rate, to a higher level and at a lesser cost than gains achieved by a "control" group in the more traditional resource room model typically utilized for students requiring special help. (Sarff, Ray, and Bagwell, 1981, p. 11.)

The cost of amplifying each classroom was $1500, whereas the cost for hiring a special education teacher and providing facilities, materials, and supplies for a resource room was estimated to be $15,000, which is ten times as much. Both minimally hearing impaired children and regular children received sound field FM treatment in classes. If a child had a hearing loss, this was not made known to other children in classes.

In a nonreverberant (0.3 to 0.4 seconds) room, a sound field FM system has the same effect upon classroom listening as moving closer to students. This was indicated recently in a study of normal hearing and minimally hard of hearing kindergarten students. Test stimuli were lists of words played back from a tape recorder. The listening treatments were: (A) sound propagation from an average of 12 feet, (B) sound propagation from an average of 4 feet, and (C) sound field FM transmission from an average of 12 feet. Suspended ceiling tiles permitted easy installation of loudspeaker tiles for the FM condition. These treatments are diagrammed in Figure 7–4.

The results indicated that (1) the normal hearing children scored significantly higher than the hard of hearing children, (2) treatments B and C resulted in significantly higher scores than treatment A, and (3) the lowest scores occurred when hard of hearing students listened without FM equipment from an average of 12 feet.

Treatment A simulates the common listening situation involving teacher and students. Under this treatment, students cannot recognize speech optimally. Treatment B demonstrates the advantage of moving closer to students. However, not all students are still able to lipread the teacher. In contrast, Treatment C is a practical solution for classroom instruction because of the S/N advantage of FM signal transmission combined with the lipreading advantage of distant listening.

Candidates for Personal FM

Personal FM provides even more S/N advantage than sound field FM. The difference may be derived from mouth-microphone distance for personal FM versus mouth-microphone plus loudspeaker-listener distance for sound field FM. A personal FM system may provide a 25+ dB S/N ratio at 12 feet. At the same distance, a sound field system may provide a 10+ dB S/N ratio. A 25+ dB S/N ratio enables a hearing aid user to listen effectively across a noisy and reverberant classroom.

When students with mild, moderate, and severe bilateral hearing losses replace their hearing aids with individual FM receivers, their speech recognition scores improve dramatically. Table 7–1 compares word recognition scores of nine hearing impaired students for hearing aid versus FM conditions. Students were seated 8 to 14 feet from a person speaking. Listening scores were consistently higher under the FM condition.

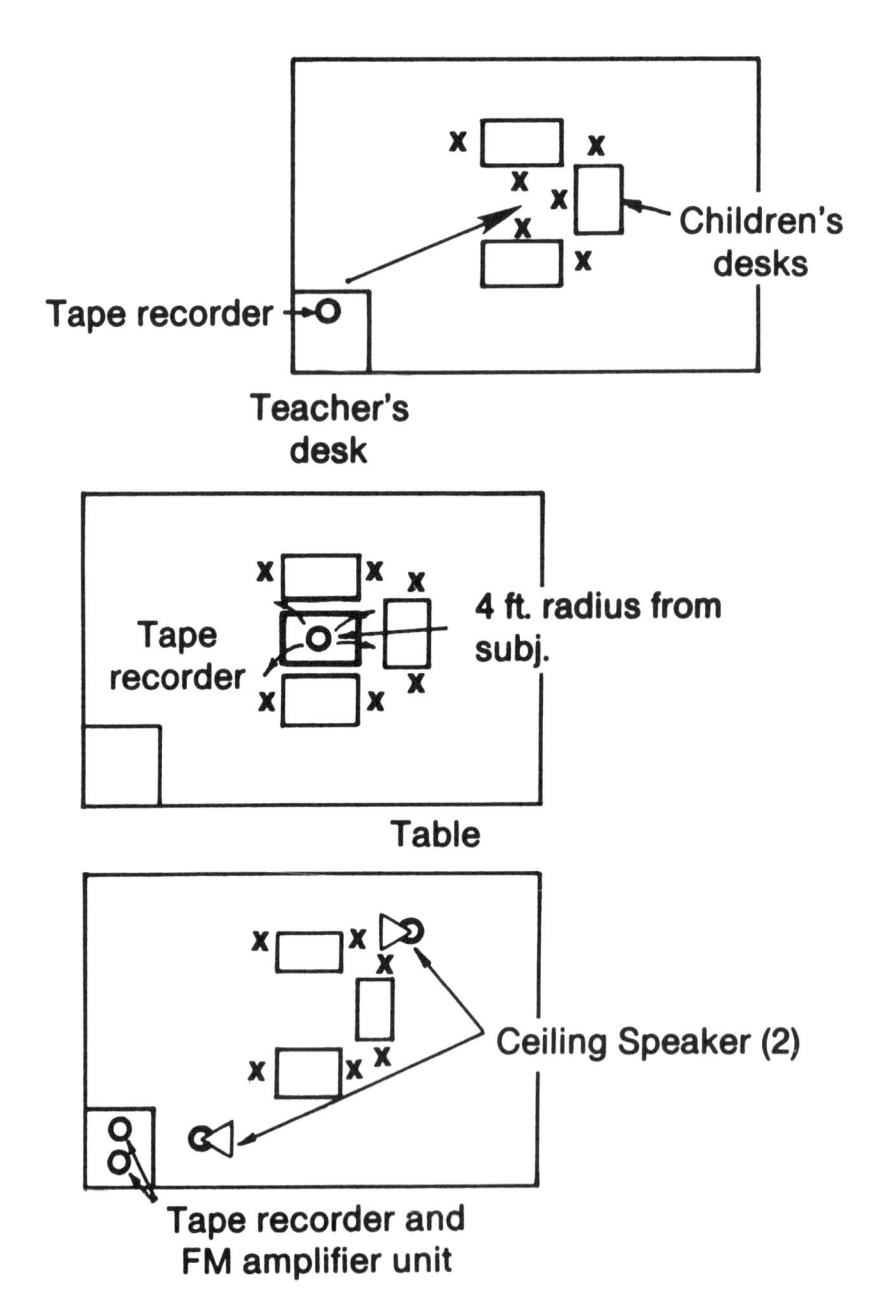

Figure 7-4. Block diagrams of three listening treatments showing sound source and children and presence or absence of FM equipment. (From Jones, J. (1986). Listening of kindergarten students under close, distant, and sound field FM amplification conditions, Ed.S. Thesis. Logan, UT: Utah State University. Reprinted by permission.)

Table 7-1. Word Recognition Percentages of Students Using Hearing Aids Versus Using Personal FM Equipment

Student	Personal FM	Hearing Aid	Difference
1	48	20	28
2	98	52	46
3	24	12	12
4	68	16	52
5	22	8	14
6	50	30	20
7	24	4	20
8	52	16	36
9	98	22	76
Mean	54	20	34

Adapted from Ross, M. (1982). *Hard of hearing children in regular schools.* Englewood Cliffs, NJ: Prentice-Hall. Copyright 1982 by Prentice-Hall, Inc. Reprinted by permission.

When hard of hearing students lipread as well as hear, they can listen more effectively in a classroom, whether using hearing aids or FM receivers. This was demonstrated in a study of auditory versus auditory-visual listening performance of hard of hearing students in noisy classrooms. Table 7-2 presents data for an "ideal" nonreverberant classroom and a typical classroom. The doors were left open and the children and teachers interacted constantly. The students repeated lists of tape recorded sentences from 1.8 meters under four treatments: (1) hearing aid, (2) hearing aid and lipreading, (3) FM transmission, and (4) FM transmission and lipreading.

Table 7-2. Auditory and Auditory-Visual Listening Performance of Hard of Hearing Students in Noisy Classroom Environments

Treatment	"Ideal" classroom (−7 dB S/N ratio) Range	Mean	"Typical" classroom (0 dB S/N ratio) Range	Mean	Total mean
Hearing aids	14–88	48	26–84	54	51
Hearing aids + lipreading	50–92	75	32–96	68	72
FM equipment	46–94	70	62–90	77	74
FM equipment + lipreading	64–94	83	66–98	88	86

Adapted from Blair, J. (1977). The effects of amplification, speechreading, and classroom environments on reception of speech. *The Volta Review, 79,* p. 447. By permission.

Table 7-3. Comparative Listening Percentages of Near Deaf and Hard of Hearing Students from 12 Feet in a Relatively Quiet and Nonreverberant Room Under Two Treatments

	Hearing + lipreading Near Deaf Students			Hearing Only Hard of hearing students			
	1	2	Mean	1	2	3	Mean
Hearing aid	40	76	58	80	100	80	87
Personal FM	78	74	76	88	100	88	92

Adapted from Berg, F., et al. *Listening in classrooms, hard of hearing.* Logan, UT: Utah State University. By permission.

Some students with profound bilateral hearing impairment use lipreading and hearing aids to try to listen in classrooms. With minimal hearing, they are particularly dependent on a high S/N ratio. Thus, personal FM equipment is preferable, although both types of FM systems are better than using a hearing aid alone. Listening scores of these near deaf students are significantly lower than those of most hard of hearing students, even when they have access to lipreading cues. Table 7–3 presents data on two near deaf students and three hard of hearing students who listened during quiet hours in a classroom that was acoustically treated. The scores of the near deaf students indicated they did not listen effectively. They had also just completed a listening training program. The scores of the hard of hearing students suggest that many hard of hearing students may listen effectively in quiet nonreverberant classrooms with either hearing aids or personal FM equipment.

COMPONENTS

To use FM equipment effectively requires understanding of FM components and accessories, and their function, operation and maintenance. A personal or sound field FM system has several basic components and some options that need to be especially considered. These will be explained in as simple terms as possible.

Microphone

A "live" voice enters an FM system via a microphone, which converts a sound signal into an electrical signal. The microphone can be nondirectional or directional in type. A nondirectional microphone is often selected for a personal FM system, and a directional microphone for a sound field FM system. An ultradirectional or noise cancelling microphone is also used. It provides the highest S/N ratio of any microphone. It is especially useful when the teacher has to talk in the vicinity of a high intensity noise.

Microphones for FM equipment are usually wearable. Other microphones are handheld. Figure 7-5 shows three wearable microphone options. The popular clip-on lavalier-style nondirectional microphone is shown with a cord attached to an FM transmitter in Figure 7-5. A self-contained directional microphone, on top of an FM transmitter, is shown in part B. A noise canceling microphone worn by a shop teacher is shown in part C.

Two handheld microphone options are pictured in Figure 7-6. A plug-in microphone is shown on the left and a boom-style microphone on the right. Each of these is directly connected to an FM transmitter. Handheld microphones are directional microphones. They are used for group participation, interviewing, or instruction in which it is desirable to pass the microphone around, or for individualized speech and listening training.

A windscreen can be used to cover a microphone. Its purpose is to keep wind noise or breathy speech sounds from interfering with signal input into the microphone. Breath noise is picked up when the mouth is held very close to the microphone.

The lavalier microphone is clipped on a shirt, a blouse, or a tie, 6 inches below the mouth of the teacher. The self-contained directional microphone FM transmitter is hung from the neck and positioned 6 inches below the mouth. The noise cancelling microphone is fastened on a headband and positioned to the side of the mouth.

A microphone is rugged, but if dropped or otherwise mishandled, it is subject to damage. If a microphone is damaged, the signal will sound distorted or noisy. It should then be replaced with a new microphone. High quality microphones for FM equipment cost from $50 to $75.

Recorded and Broadcast Signals

A microphone permits a "live" voice to enter a FM system and be transmitted to students or other listeners. Recorded and broadcast sound signals can also be transmitted through an FM system. A cassette recorder, stereo, TV, radio, or other audio source of signals can be electrically connected to an FM transmitter. In some FM systems, the microphone and recorded or broadcast sound sources are both connected to the transmitter. A squelch circuit permits the "live" signal to override the other signal, if both enter simultaneously.

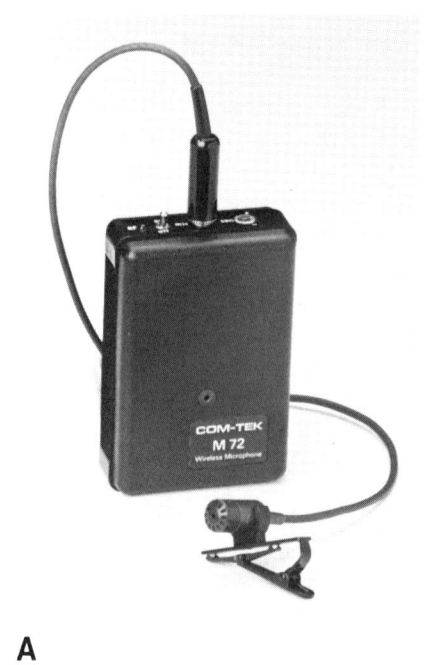

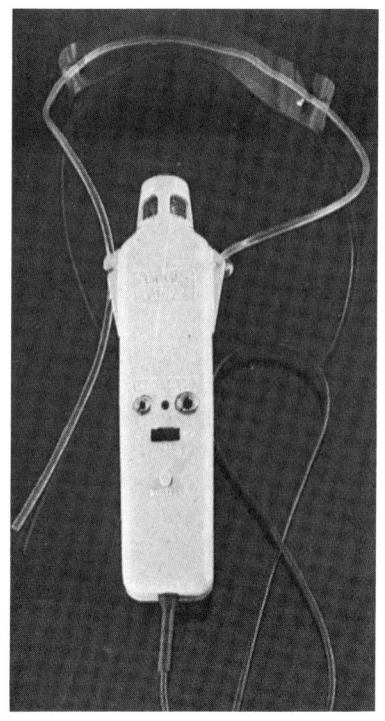

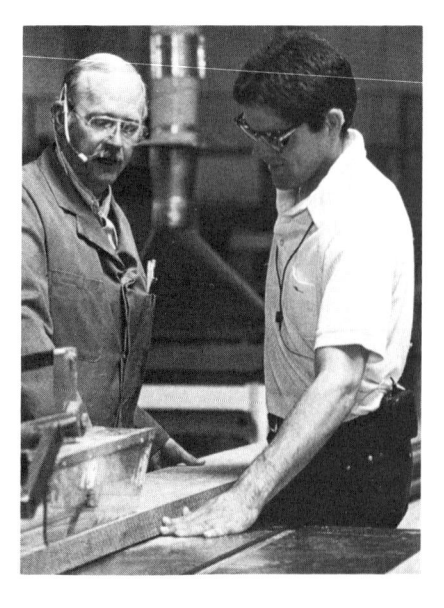

Figure 7-5. Wearable microphone options for FM equipment. (A, C) Non directional lavalier and noise cancelling microphones (From COMTEK advertisement flyer. Salt Lake City: Communications Technology, Inc. Reprinted by permission.) (B) Directional microphone (From TELEX advertisement flyer. Minneapolis: Telex Communications, Inc. Reprinted by permission.)

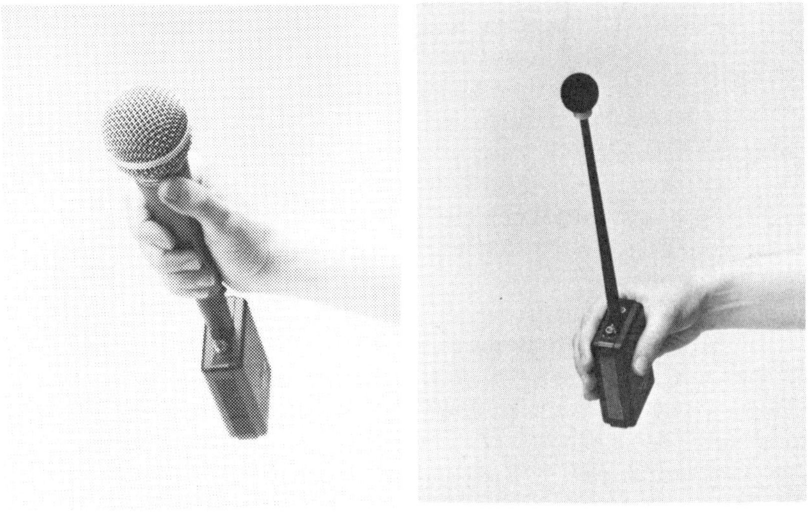

FM Equipment   167

Figure 7-6. Handheld microphone options connected to an FM transmitter. (From COMTEK advertisement flyer. Salt Lake City: Communications Technology, Inc. Reprinted by permission.)

In a classroom, the signal that enters the FM transmitter is usually the teacher's voice. There are occasions, however, when it is desirable for students to listen to a radio, TV, audio cassette recording, video cassette recording, or even sound track of a motion picture. These audio sources can be heard better when transmitted through an FM system. When a recorded or broadcast sound is heard without being transmitted, it attenuates over distance, and noise and reverberation interfere with hearing it. Patch cords can be purchased to interconnect audio sources and an FM transmitter. A teacher should know how to operate audio equipment and to interconnect it with the transmitter.

Audiovisual (AV) equipment services in a school or community can assist a teacher with recording and broadcast accessories. This equipment is relatively inexpensive and can be shared by teachers in a school. It is often located in school media and library centers. Teachers may also have their own AV equipment. A combination radio and cassette recorder, which can be purchased for less than $50, is often owned by a teacher. This combines both recorded and broadcast sound signals.

Transmitter

An FM transmitter is the most expensive component of an FM system. It includes provision for input of "live," recorded, or broadcast signals. The transmitter also includes a subcomponent that produces radio signals, a subcomponent that moduulates radio signals with audio signals, a battery, and an antenna from which the radio wave is transmitted. The antenna can be within the transmitter or extend from it.

The FM signal is transmitted at a radio frequency assigned by the Federal Communications Commission (FCC) for assistive listening transmission applications. The number of frequencies assigned for FM equipment used by the hearing impaired depends on the locality. Each classroom has to have a different radio frequency or channel. The frequency of each transmitter is determined during its manufacture. The transmitter has to be returned to the factory if the frequency is to be changed.

Only one FM transmitter on the same channel can be used at the same time in a classroom. If another transmitter is added, a chirping sound will result. If still additional FM transmitters are used simultaneously in the same classroom, none of their signals will be understood. This means that only one person can transmit a signal on the same channel at one time, although many persons can listen to this signal simultaneously. The transmitter with attached microphone has to be passed from the teacher to others if they are to transmit their voices.

An FM transmitter is often attached to a belt. A transmitter worn at this position is connected to an external microphone positioned under the chin. An FM transmitter may also be suspended from the neck. Figure 7–7 shows these two popular options.

Rough handling can damage an FM transmitter. Some companies provide carrying pouches to protect transmitters. Belt pouches cost very little and should be used when available.

In a school auditorium or other large room with a public address (PA) system, an FM transmitter can be installed. The transmitter is connected into the PA system with an adapter unit. The transmitter is also plugged into a wall circuit so that a battery does not have to be used. With this arrangement, the signal from the PA system can be transmitted to students using FM receivers. Otherwise, students have to listen to the PA system from ceiling loudspeakers, providing a poor S/N ratio. Figure 7–8 shows an FM transmitter and adapter unit, with an upward extending antenna.

Receiver

An FM receiver is the counterpart to an FM transmitter. A personal FM receiver includes an antenna, which intercepts the FM transmitted signal, a demodulator, which separates the audio signal from the radio signal, an amplifier, and listener coupler or hearing aid. A sound field FM receiver also includes an antenna, a demodulator, and an amplifier. It is coupled to loudspeakers to enhance group listening.

FM Equipment   169

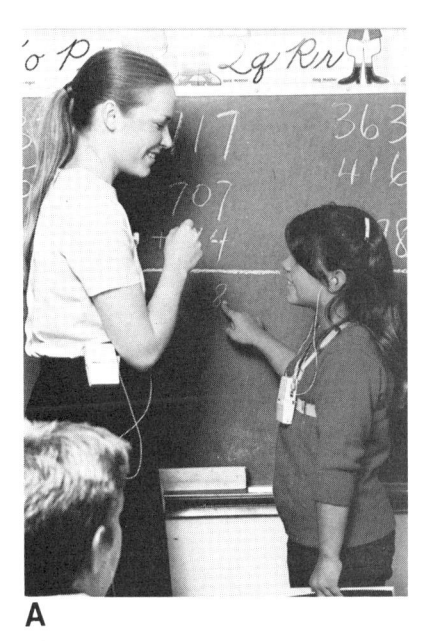

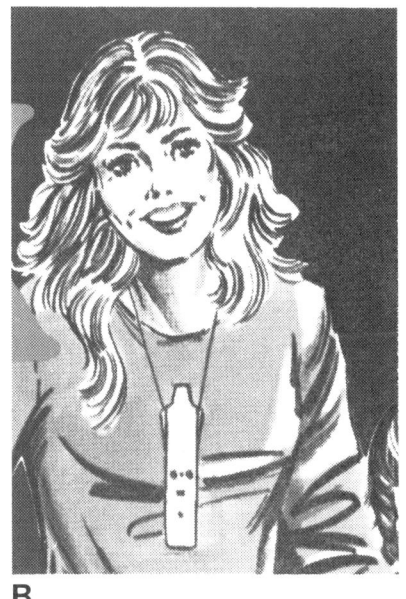

Figure 7-7. (A) A teacher with a belt-worn transmitter. (From Phonic Ear advertisement flyer. Mill Valley, CA: Phonic Ear, Inc. Reprinted by permission.) (B) A teacher with a suspended microphone. (From Telex advertisement flyer. Minneapolis: Telex Communications, Inc. Reprinted by permission.)

An FM receiver is tuned to the channel frequency transmitted from an FM transmitter. Most FM receivers use plug-in crystal modules. Each module is tuned to a different frequency. Plug-in crystal modules make it easy for a listener to change receiver channels in moving from one classroom to another. When purchased, the FM receiver and transmitter are channel matched. Specific frequency channels are designated by letters and numbers. A less expensive but more inflexible arrangement is internal adjustment of frequency rather than switching of crystal modules. Figure 7-9 shows a crystal module being plugged into an FM receiver.

Any number of FM receivers can be used simultaneously in the same classroom if they are on the same channel. Hearing impaired students using these receivers can be located anywhere. Figure 7-10 shows three young students using personal FM receivers and a teacher using an FM transmitter.

An FM receiver can also include a monaural or binaural hearing aid. This feature permits the user to listen to a radio signal from the FM

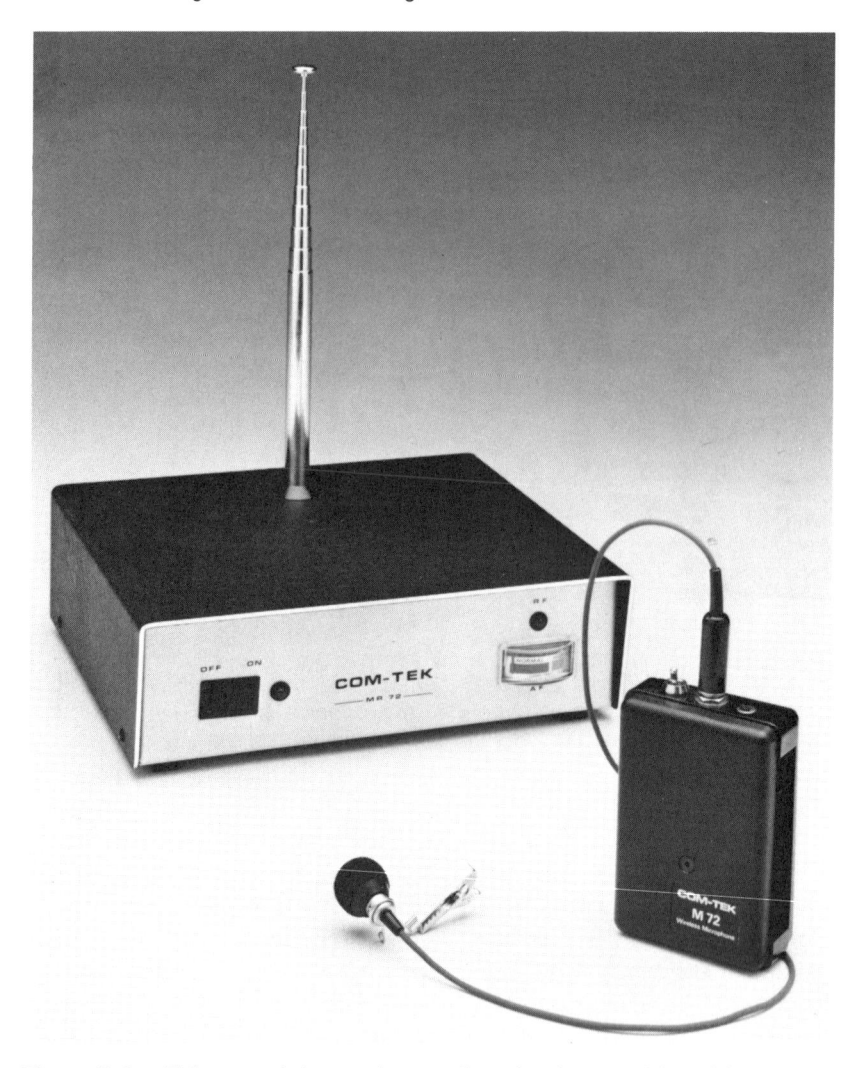

Figure 7-8. FM transmitting equipment for adapting a public address system. (From COMTEK advertisement flyer. Salt Lake City: Communications Technology, Inc. Reprinted by permission.)

transmitter, a sound signal through one or two microphones, or both in combination. When the FM receiver includes a hearing aid, the unit is attached to the chest of the listener to enhance environmental sound reception. When the FM receiver does not include a hearing aid, it is usually attached to the listener's belt (Fig. 7–11). A belt pouch is recommended to protect the receiver from damage.

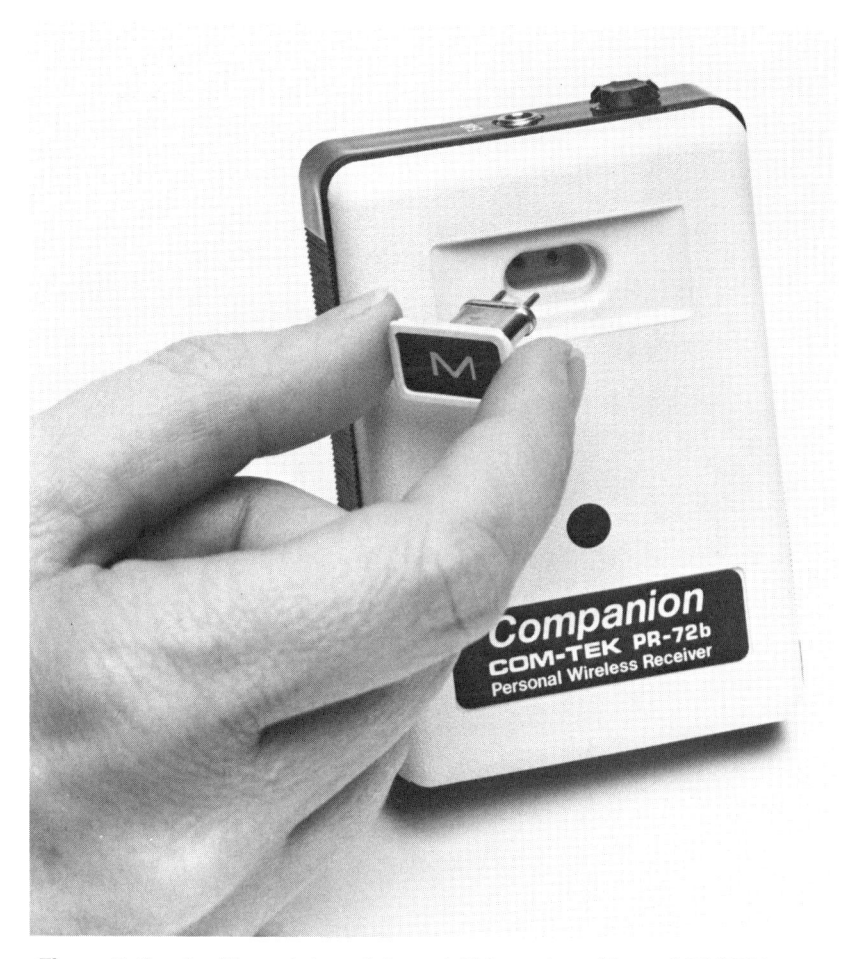

Figure 7-9. An M crystal module and FM receiver (From COMTEK advertisement flyer. Salt Lake City: Communications Technology, Inc. Reprinted by permission.)

Some school districts purchase hearing aids in FM receivers for young hearing impaired students. Combined FM–hearing aid units are referred to as student receivers. Owning the units gives the school more control over the listening of students. Caregivers do not always ensure that a student has a functioning hearing aid.

A personal FM receiver basically provides amplification for the audio signal that has been separated from the radio signal. It also couples this signal directly to a miniaturized earphone assembly or headset, or to a student's own hearing aid. If the student is using two

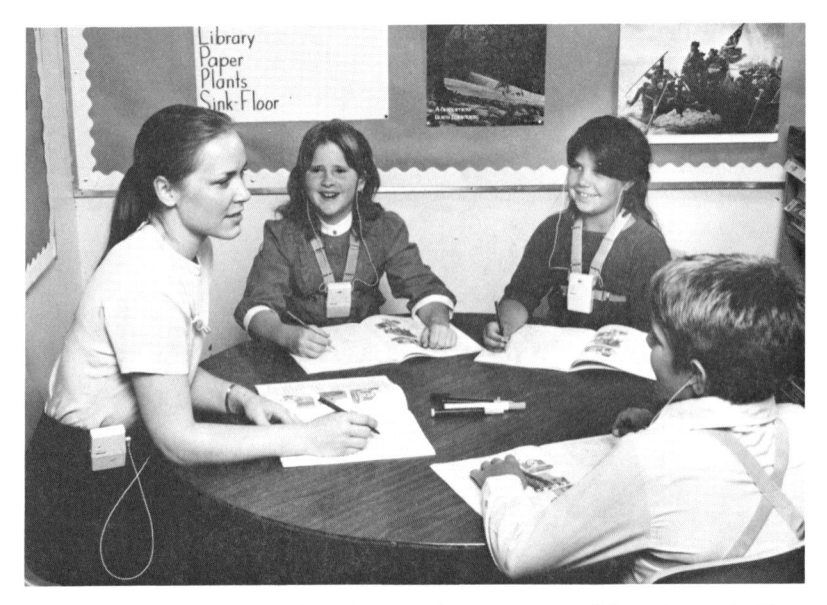

Figure 7-10. Teacher and students using personal FM equipment. (From Phonic Ear advertisement flyer. Mill Valley, CA: Phonic Ear, Inc. Reprinted by permission.)

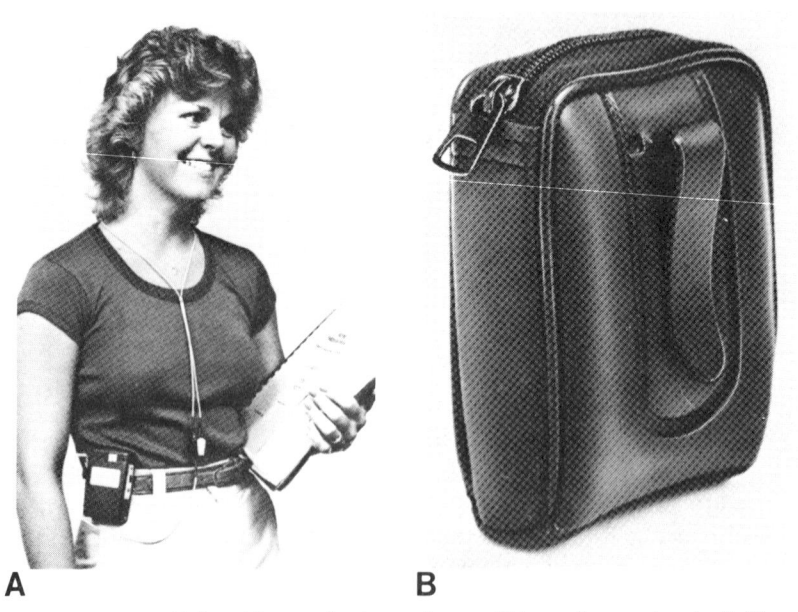

A B

Figure 7-11. (A) An older student wearing an FM receiver on her belt. (From Telex advertisement flyer. Minneapolis: Telex Communications, Inc. Reprinted by permission.) (B) A belt pouch. (From COMTEK advertisement flyer. Salt Lake City: Communications Technology, Inc. Reprinted by permission.)

earphones or wearing binaural hearing aids, the signal goes to both ears. It is preferable to have students use their own hearing aids for two reasons. First, their aids have been already matched to their unique hearing losses. Second, the parents become involved in providing continuity of listening between the home and school. Personal FM systems that incorporate hearing aids have enough fitting flexibility to meet the needs of many, but not all, hearing impaired children. Figure 7-12 shows a binaural student receiver with gain, output, and frequency response controls.

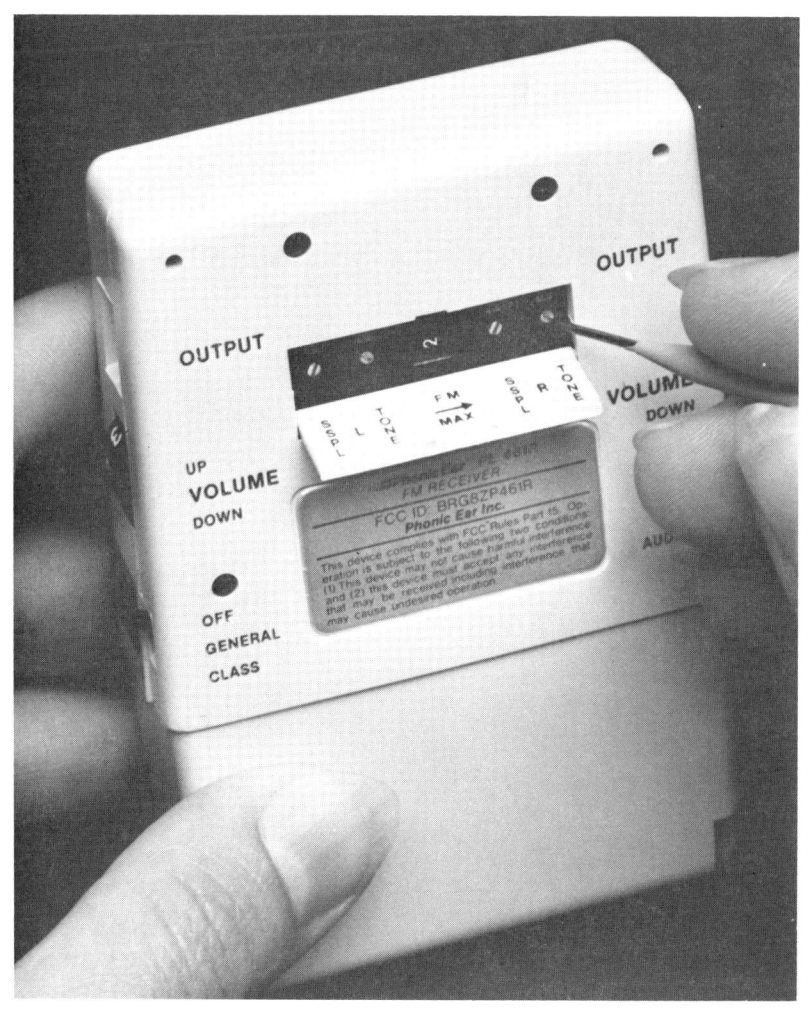

Figure 7-12. FM student receiver with trimmer controls for individual fitting. (From Phonic Ear advertisement flyer. Mill Valley, CA: Phonic Ear, Inc. Reprinted by permission.)

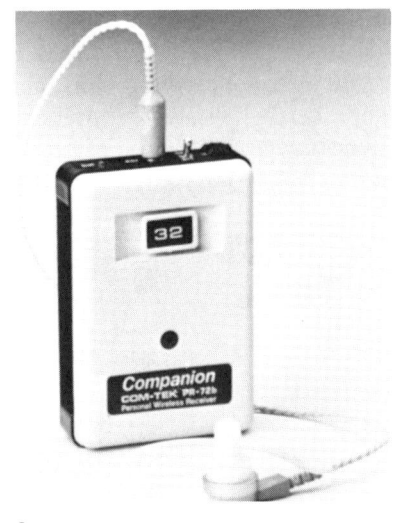

Figure 7–13. FM receiver options. (A) Direct input to earphone assembly. (B) Direct input to hearing aid. (C) Magnetic input to hearing aid. (From COMTEK advertisement flyer. Salt Lake City, UT: Communications Technology, Inc. Reprinted by permission.

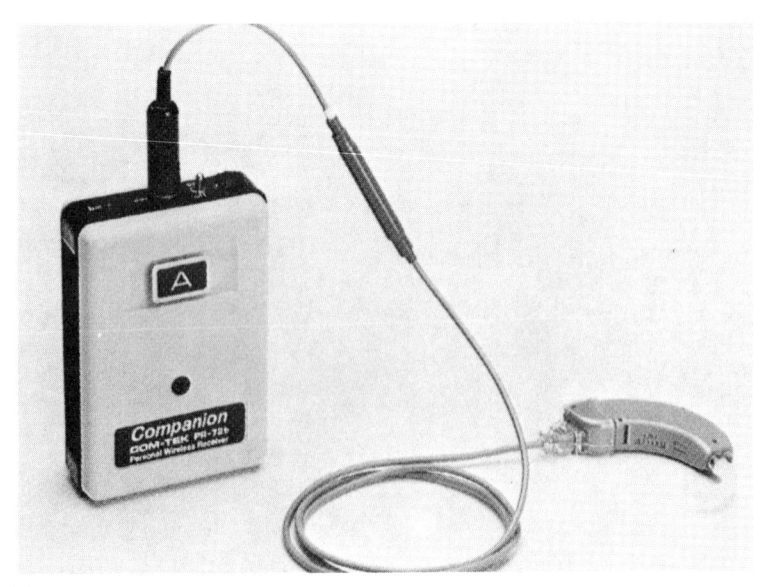

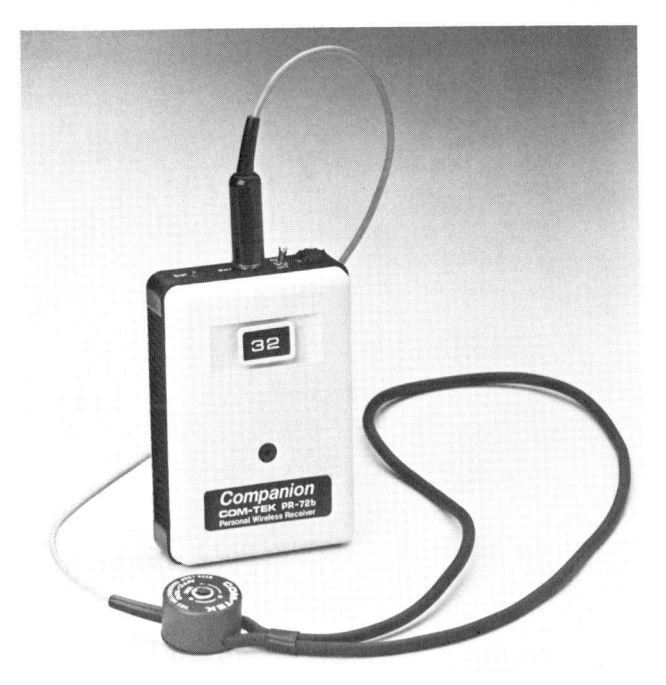

C

Three FM receiver output options are available: (1) direct wire to earphone assembly, (2) direct wire to BTE hearing aid, and (3) magnetic input to BTE or ITE hearing aid. The first option is used if the FM receiver has a built-in hearing aid. The earphone assembly serves as the receiver of the hearing aid, transducing the amplified electrical signal into an amplified sound signal. This option is also used with a basic FM receiver for a student with a minimal hearing loss or for a teacher who is checking the FM system.

The second output option is used with hearing aids that have a special plug-in. The third option may be used with hearing aids that have a telecoil. A magnetic loop is worn around the neck of the student. With the aid of the loop, the signal from the FM receiver is converted into a magnetic signal, which induces an electrical signal in the hearing aid telecoil. Figure 7-13 shows these output options.

When the student's own hearing aid is used, it is debatable whether to use a plug-in or a magnetic loop and telecoil. The plug-in seems preferable because it involves fewer energy conversions and may be less distorted. Many students, however, prefer magnetic input because the magnetic loop can be concealed under an outer garment. Both options

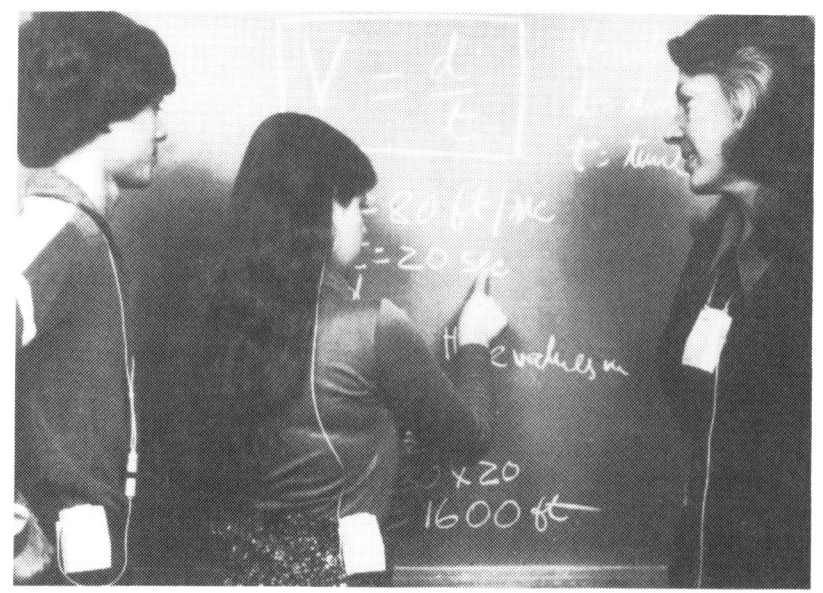

A

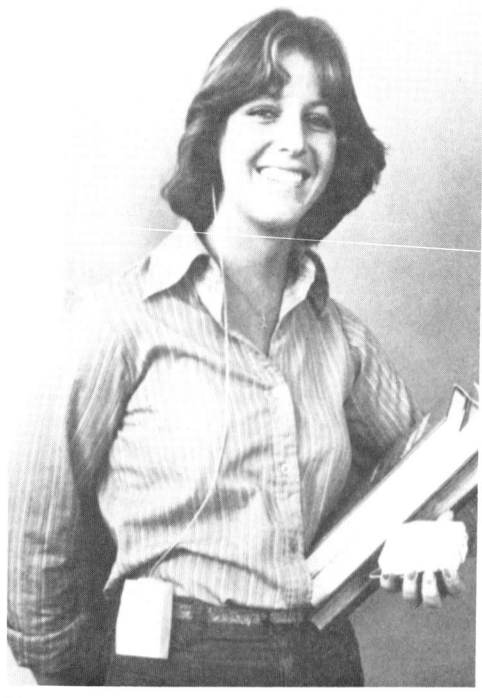

B

Figure 7-14. (A) Two students using FM receiver with magnetic loops. Ordinarily the cords would be concealed. (B) A student using an FM receiver with a direct input to a hearing aid. The connecting wire is visible but the hearing aid is concealed by the student's hair. (From Phonic Ear advertisement flyer. Mill Valley, CA: Phonic Ear, Inc. Reprinted by permission.)

can result in speech recognition scores comparable to those obtained in a hearing test booth. These input options to hearing aids are shown in Figure 7–14.

When a sound field FM receiver, amplifier, and loudspeakers are used, the sound output in decibels and the frequency response can be controlled. For example, the amplifier output may be given high frequency emphasis to enhance speech recognition. The receiver, amplifier, and loudspeakers have a very wide frequency response and high internal S/N ratio to enhance student listening. Figure 7–15 includes photographs of the amplifier and of responding students. Loudspeakers are positioned on either the ceiling or floor to enhance projection of sound toward the class. The FM receiver is not shown but is positioned beside or on top of the amplifier.

Batteries

Personal FM transmitters and receivers are powered by 9 volt batteries. Alkaline or nickel cadmium batteries may be used. Alkaline batteries last for approximately 30 hours. Nickel cadmium batteries may be recharged for years. Various battery chargers are available. The chargers are powered by wall circuit current. Figure 7–16 shows alkaline batteries in FM transmitter and receiver units and a battery charger.

OPERATION

The operation of FM equipment will now be described. Personal FM equipment manufactured by Comtek will be featured. The operation of equipment and accessories from other companies is similar. Comtek personal FM components and accessories are shown in Figure 7–17. With study and hands-on experience with this kit, a teacher will learn how to use personal FM equipment. This information has been developed basically by Ralph Belgigue, President and Chief Engineer of Comtek.

Teachers should first demonstrate to themselves the operation of the FM transmitter and receiver units found in the kit.

Transmitter Unit

The cord for the microphone and clip is plugged into the jack in the top of the transmitter. The switch next to the jack is next turned on. Clip the microphone to your belt so the signal is not too intense when you talk.

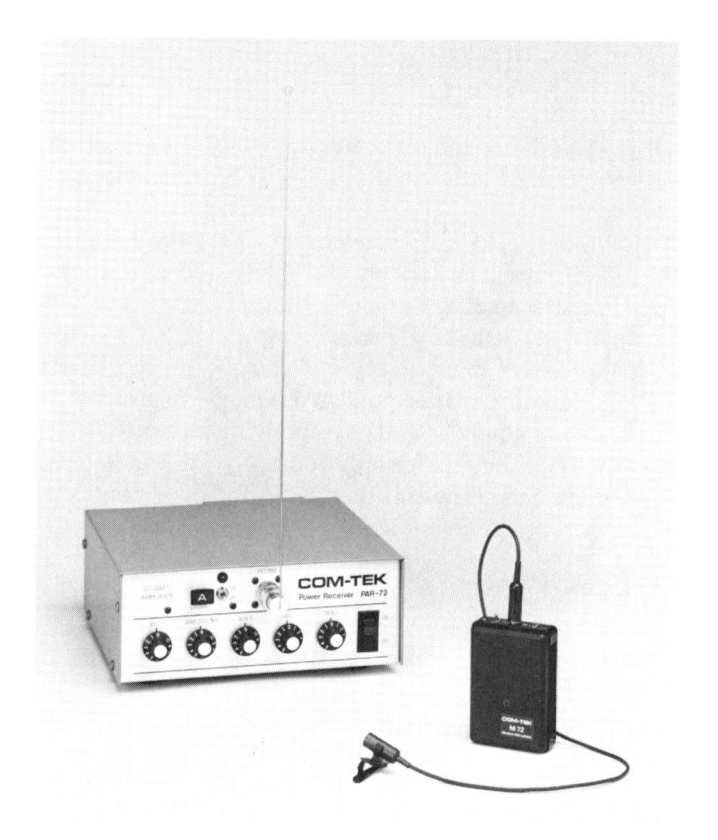

A

B

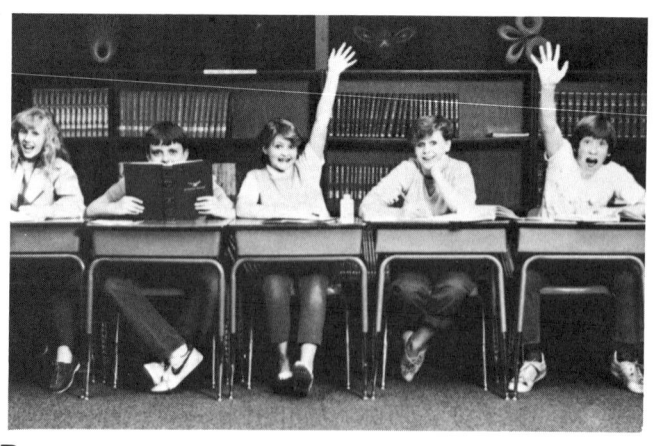

Figure 7-15. Sound field FM equipment. (A) A lavalier microphone, transmitter, receiver, and amplifier. (B) Students responding to an FM transmitted and loudspeaker (not shown) delivered signal from a teacher. (From Omni-2000 advertisement flyer. Orem, UT: Audio Enhancement Systems. Reprinted by permission.)

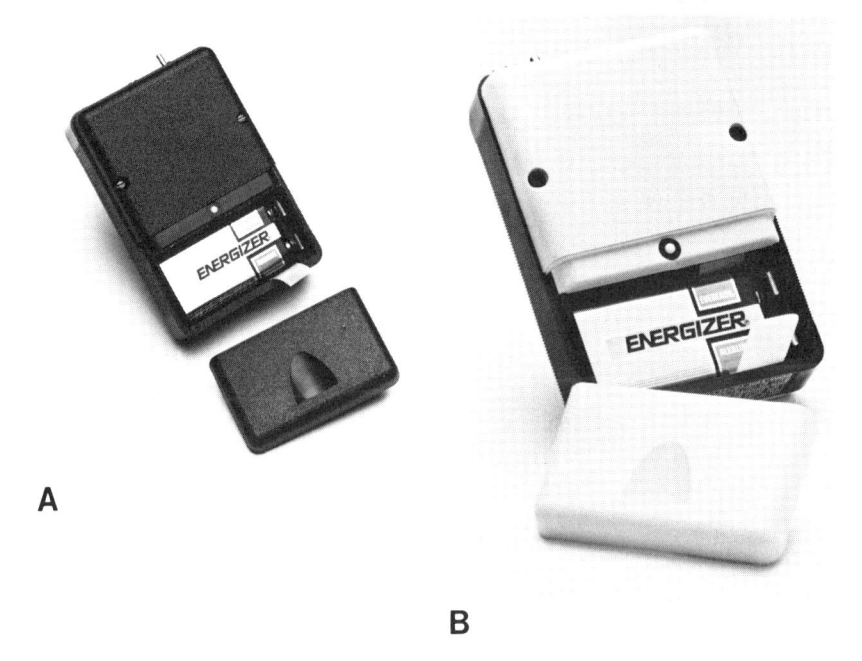

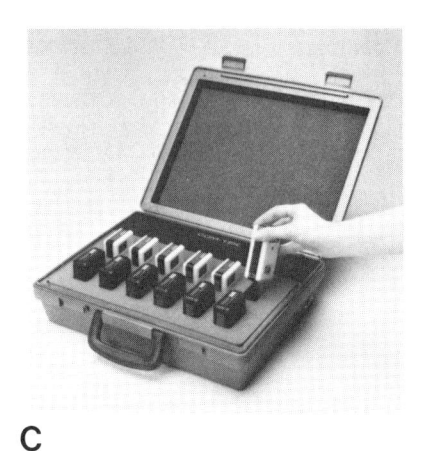

Figure 7-16. Battery equipment. (A) Battery in transmitter, (B) battery in receiver, and (C) 12-unit charger/carrying case. (From Com Tek advertisement flyers. Salt Lake City: Communications Technology, Inc. Reprinted by permission.)

Receiver Unit

The cord for the earphone assembly is plugged into the jack in the top of the receiver. The earphone assembly should be plugged in your ear. The volume control next to the receiver jack should be rotated counterclockwise so that sound is not to loud when you speak. Now, talk and listen.

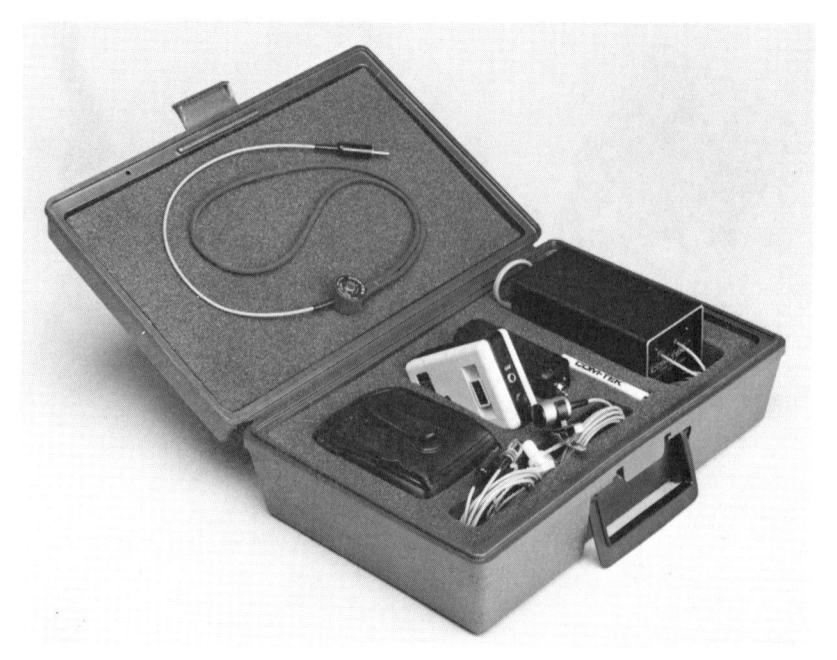

Figure 7-17. Personal FM carrying case. Equipment includes transmitter (M-72-AT), personal receiver (PR-72b option 1) (alkaline batteries are included and installed), rechargeable batteries (Varta 9-100), battery charger (NBC 9-2), earphone assembly (SM-N), neckloop transductor (NTC-102), microphone and clip (M-4005), accessory attenuator (CB-48), and two belt pouches (P-1's). (From Belgique, R. Wising up to your companion: Instructions for operating your Comtek AT-72. Salt Lake City: Communications Technology, Inc. Reprinted by permission.)

Recording Speech

Using the receiver, you can simultaneously (1) listen to and (2) tape record and play back your speech. The tape recording is excellent because of the high S/N ratio. The attenuator cable is used. Insert the black plug into the microphone jack of the cassette recorder. Insert the red plug into the receiver. Insert the earphone assembly plug or neck loop transductor plug into the silver jack of the attenuator adapter cable. Figure 7-18 shows this arrangement, with a neck loop transductor cable appropriate for a hearing aid user.

Transmitting Recorded Speech or Music

The attenuator adapter cable can also be used to transmit from a tape recorder, stereo, TV, radio, or other audio source instead of a "live" talker. Insert the black plug into the transmitter. Insert the red plug into

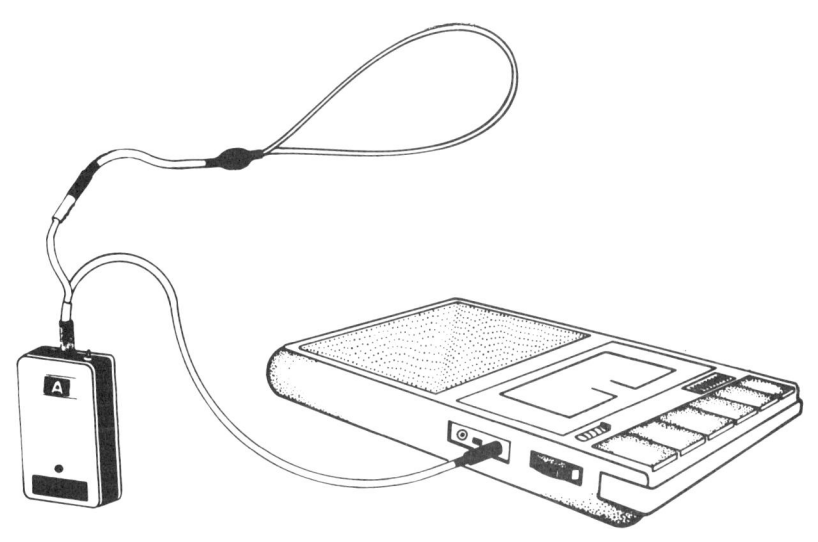

Figure 7-18. A neck loop for magnetic input to a hearing aid is plugged into an attenuator adapter cable. One plug of the cable is inserted into an FM receiver and the other into a cassette recorder. (From Belgigue, R. Wising up to your companion: Instructions for operating your Comtek AT-72. Salt Lake City: Communications Technology, Inc. Reprinted by permission.)

the output of the audio source. Figure 7-19 illustrates these connections. In the instance of the cassette recorder, the recorded signal will now be transmitted to the person using the receiver.

A teacher can next demonstrate the FM transmitter and receiver units with a person using a hearing aid. Both magnetic input and direct input to a hearing aid will be described. An auxiliary cord is supplied with a BTE hearing aid adapted for direct input.

Transmitter Unit

Follow the same procedures as you did when you demonstrated the transmitter on yourself. However, clip the microphone to your shirt pocket rather than your belt, since the speech signal can be more intense.

Receiver Unit and Magnetic Input

The cord for the neck loop transductor is plugged into the jack in the top of the receiver. The loop should be placed around the neck of the person wearing a BTE aid. It can be under the shirt and not show. The volume of the hearing aid should provide a comfortable loudness level as you speak,

Monitoring output jack

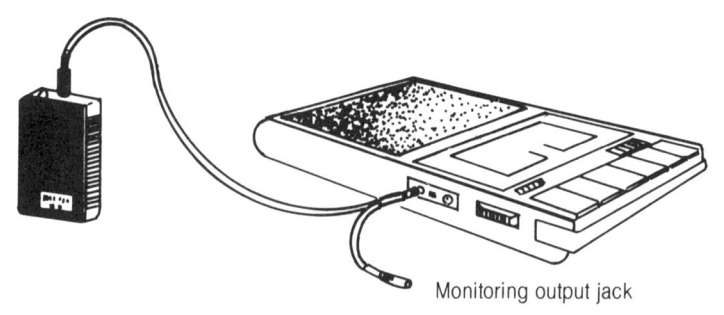

Figure 7-19. An attenuator adapter cable hook up for transmitting a tape recording from an FM transmitter. (From Belgigue, R. Wising up to your companion: Instructions for operating your Comtek AT-72. Salt Lake City: Communications Technology, Inc. Reprinted by permission.)

with the aid turned to the M (microphone) position. Switch the aid to the T (telecoil) position, speak and determine if the sound volume is comfortable for the person. Adjust the volume control on the receiver to the most comfortable loudness level for the hearing aid user. Now alternate between the M and T positions of the hearing aid while speaking, and adjust the volume on the receiver until it is about equal in both settings. Walk away from the hearing aid user and continue to speak at a normal loudness level. Your speech may be heard no matter where you are located within 200 feet. Figure 7-20 pictures a four position control for switching from off to microphone-telephone, telephone, or microphone use on a hearing aid. It also shows an FM receiver with neck loop transductor for magnetic input.

Receiver Unit and Direct Input

One end of a line cord for a BTE hearing aid is plugged in the top of the FM receiver. The other end is plugged into a "shoe," which is plugged into the aid. Figure 7-21 shows an Oticon aid, shoe, and line cord. A hearing aid company will supply a cord with a terminal that is compatible for a company's FM receiver. This aid has a screwdriver adjustable control that can be set for a desired sound balance between FM equipment (teacher's voice) and the hearing aid's microphone (surrounding sounds). Leave the volume control of the hearing aid where the user has it. Set the balance control of the aid to a high S/N ratio. While speaking, adjust the volume control of the FM receiver to the most comfortable loudness level for the hearing aid user. Walk up to 1200 feet away from the hearing aid user and you will still be heard.

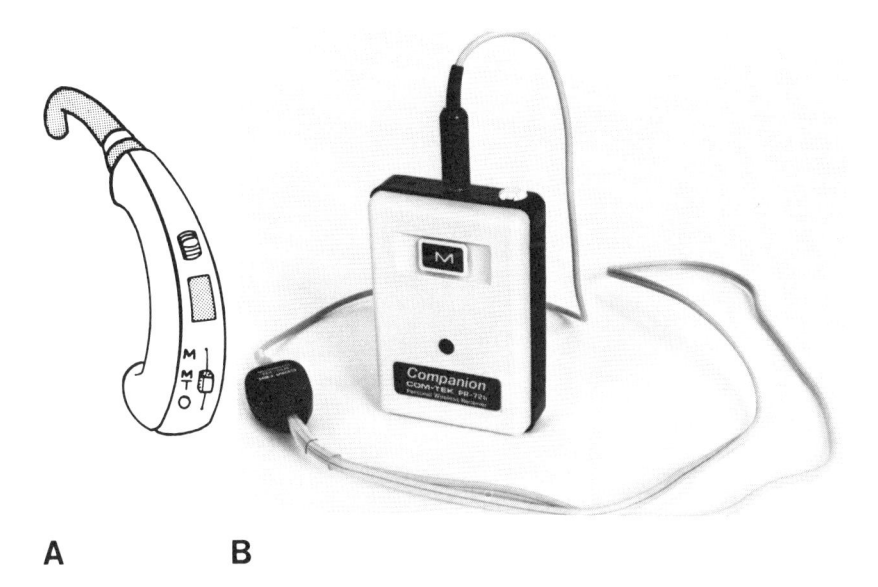

Figure 7-20. (A) A behind-the-ear aid with a four position off-microphone-microphone-telephone switch. (From Belgigue, R. Wising up to your companion: Instructions for operating your Comtek AT-72. (B) An FM receiver with a neck loop transductor. Salt Lake City: Communications Technology, Inc. Reprinted by permission.)

Batteries

Alkaline batteries are already in the transmitter and receiver units. They may be replaced after 30 hours of use or recharged to a limited extent. Nickel cadmium (VARTA) batteries are included in the Comtek kit. They can be used for 6 hours but then need to be recharged for at least 12 hours. To insert a battery, slide open the battery compartment located on the back of the transmitter or receiver. Match the battery terminals marked (+)(−) with the (+)(−) on the label of the battery compartment. Press the battery into the compartment by placing the bottom of the battery in position first. The battery pull tab should be underneath the battery when installed.

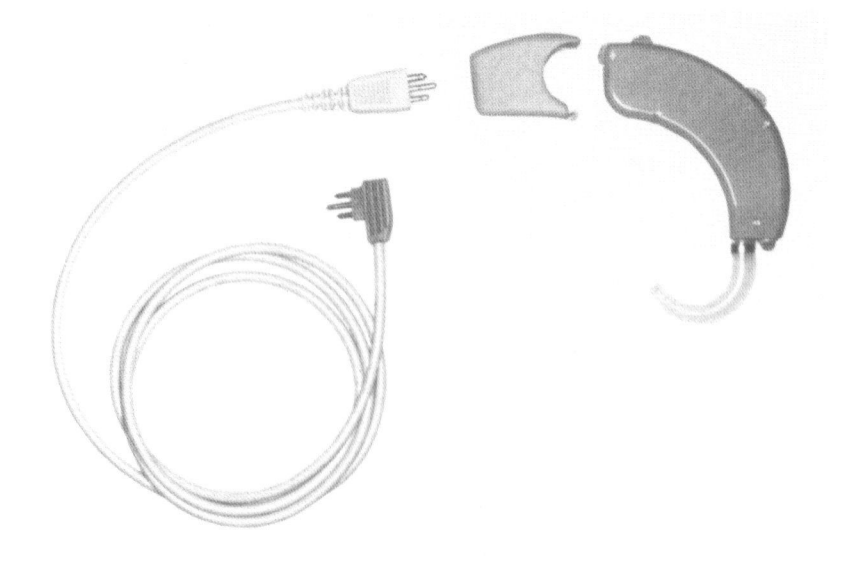

A

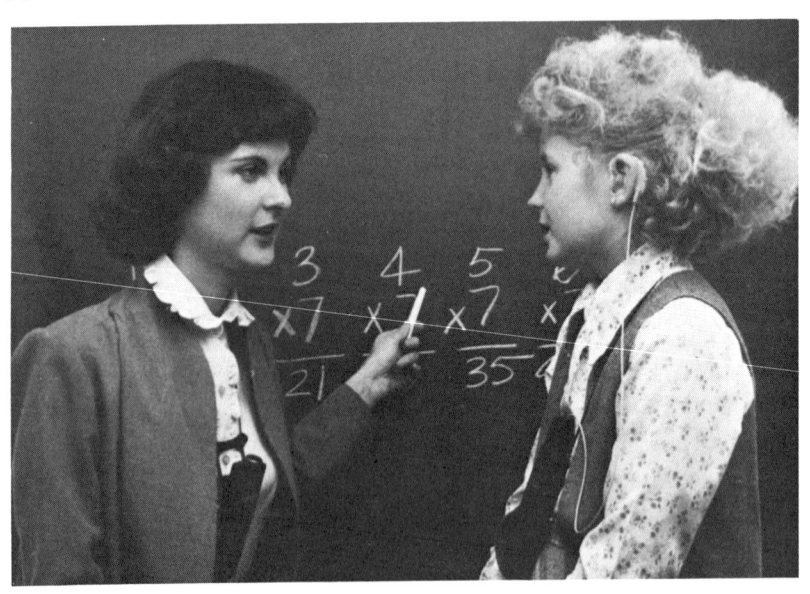

B

Figure 7-21. (A) A line cord shoe and BTE aid. From Oticon advertisement. Somerset, NJ: Oticon Corporation. Reprinted by permission. (B) A teacher using a direct input aid. From Unitron advertisement. Port Huron, MI: Unitron Industries, Inc. Reprinted by permission.

Battery Charger

To recharge the transmitter or receiver's nickel cadmium batteries, (1) plug the battery charger into any 110 volt outlet, (2) turn the transmitter or receiver off, and (3) insert one jack plug of the battery charger into the transmitter's microphone input (jack at top) and the other plug into the output jack at the top of the receiver. The red lights on the battery charger will glow when the charger is operating. Allow at least 12 hours to bring the batteries to full charge. This procedure may be repeated 1000 times, without need of replacing the nickel cadmium batteries. Before first use, the nickel cadmium batteries must be charged for 14 hours.

Other adjustments and features of personal FM equipment relate to the receiver crystal transmitter and receiver covers, transmitter switch and lights.

Crystal

The crystal plug-in module is located on the front of the receiver. It can be removed and replaced with another crystal. This procedure is necessary when the user moves to another classroom where another teacher is using an FM transmitter. Each teacher in a school should stock crystals for different frequency channels used by students. The M crystal shown in Figure 7–22 is one of eight frequency modules indicated by alphabet letters. The 32 crystal is one of many modules indicated by numbers.

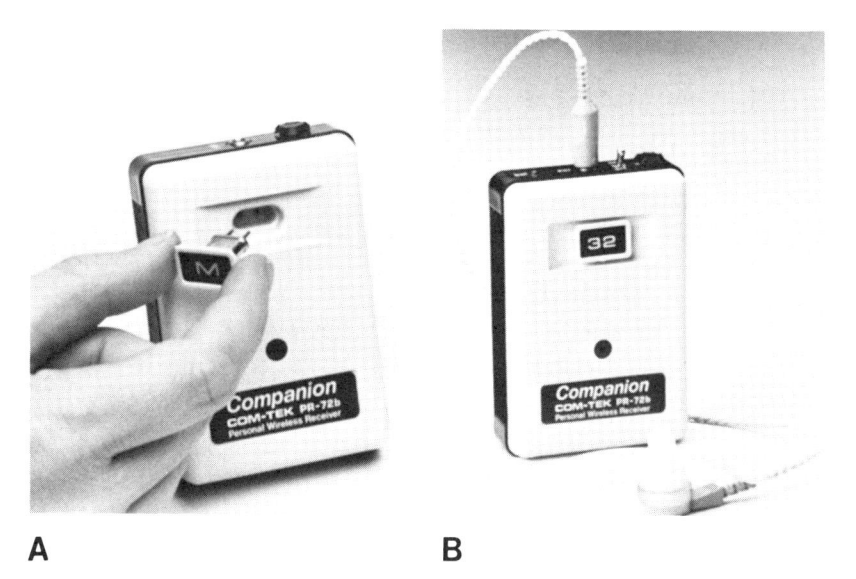

Figure 7–22. (A) The changing of a channel selector crystal. (B) A different channel selected inserted in an FM receiver. (From Comtek advertisement flyers. Salt Lake City: Communications Technology, Inc. Reprinted by permission.)

Covers

Other adjustments should be left to the factory, including removing the front and back covers of the transmitter and receiver units. Even the battery compartment can be left closed, since nickel cadmium batteries will ordinarily be used. The front cover of an FM receiver is seen in Figure 7–22.

Switch and Lights

An on-off switch is used only with the transmitter unit. The receiver unit is on when a cord is plugged into it. A red light on top of the transmitter or receiver comes on when either unit is operating.

EVALUATION AND MAINTENANCE

The evaluation and maintenance of FM equipment is necessary to ensure that children listen effectively in classrooms. Before purchasing, FM equipment should be carefully evaluated. After equipment is purchased, it should be periodically evaluated, closely maintained, and systematically serviced. Initially, school personnel should write or telephone companies for equipment information. Representatives should be asked to visit schools to explain and demonstrate equipment. Names, addresses, and telephone numbers of companies manufacturing FM equipment are listed in Table 7–4.

Once purchased, FM equipment is under short-term warranty. Companies also provide continuing repair and service. Screening for problems and minor servicing is done by local representatives or through telephone communication with company service departments. The user should take the following precautions:

Table 7-4. Companies Manufacturing FM Equipment

Comtek Communications Technology, 357 W 2700 S, Salt Lake City, UT 84115 (801) 466-3463
Earmark, 1125 Dixwell Ave., Hamden, CT 06514, (203) 777-2130
Phonic Ear, 250 Camino Alto, Mill Valley, CA 94941, (414) 383-4000
Telex Communications, 9600 Aldrich Ave., S., Minneapolis, MN 55420, (800) 328-8212
Unitron Industries, 1414 Pine Grove Ave., Port Huron, MI 48060, (800) 521-5400
Williams Sound, 6844 Washington Ave. S., Eden Prairie, MN 55344, (612) 941-2896

1. *Avoid excessive heat.* Don't leave a transmitter or a receiver in hot sun, on a radiator, or near sources of high temperature.
2. *Avoid rough handling.* The receiver and transmitter may be damaged if dropped. When possible, use protective pouches.
3. *Remove batteries* when storing a unit for a long time. When a battery becomes exhausted, it may leak and damage the instrument. Even a new battery may leak because of slight imperfections. Therefore, occasionally check them for leakage.
4. *Keep battery terminals and contacts clean.* Inspect them to ensure that they are not corroded. If they are, polish them with a pencil eraser.
5. *Inspect cord and connectors* frequently—they are subject to wear. Replace frayed cords before they break.

Initial and periodic evaluation of FM equipment can be done by an audiologist or a teacher. The audiologist can obtain detection thresholds and speech recognition scores on students in a hearing testing booth, without a hearing aid, with a hearing aid, and with FM equipment under consideration. A teacher can present "live" or recorded word or sentence lists in the classroom setting under similar conditions. Comparative word or sentence recognition scores can be obtained.

James Blair developed six sentence lists for his doctoral study at Northwestern University. These lists are included in his 1976 unpublished doctoral dissertation, entitled *The Contributing Influences of Amplification, Speechreading and Classroom Environments on the Ability of Hard of Hearing Chidren to Discriminate Sentences.*

The lists are included in Appendix A at the end of this chapter. Each sentence in a list includes two key words. This is exemplifed in the first sentence of one of the lists. The *bean* is in the *jar.* Twenty-five sentences and 50 words are in the list. Therefore, each key word counts 2 percent. Students write down or repeat the sentences a teacher says. The student is not allowed to look at the teacher unless "deaf." A percent score for each list is calculated. Each list takes 3 to 5 minutes to administer. The sentences are at the third grade level.

The Ling five sound test can also be used to evaluate FM equipment as well as hearing aids at various teacher-student distances. If a student cannot do as well with FM equipment in the classroom as with a hearing aid in a hearing testing booth, the FM equipment is of questionable benefit. Students who indicate they can hear the five sounds in the test booth should also indicate they hear the sounds from any location in a classroom when using FM equipment. Likewise, a student who obtains an 80 percent sentence recognition score in the test booth should score as well in the classroom.

SUMMARY

FM equipment is valuable for classroom listening. It compensates for distance, noise, and reverberation problems. Normal hearing students and especially hearing impaired students benefit. Both sound field and personal types of FM are assistive listening devices. Many components and accessories contribute to FM technology. Detailed study of the operation of FM equipment is needed. Evaluation procedures and maintenance guidelines should be followed.

FURTHER READINGS

Mar Ross's book *Hard of Hearing Children in Regular Schools* (Prentice-Hall, Englewood Cliffs, NJ, 1982) provides a strong case for the use of personal FM equipment in the schools. An article by Louis Sarff, Helen Ray, and Alice Bagwell in the October 1981 issue of the *Hearing Aid Journal* (volume 11, pp. 44, 47–48, 50, 52) explains why sound field FM equipment should also be used. James Blair's 1977 article in the *Volta Review* (volume 7, pp. 443–449) documents the contribution of FM signal transmission and lipreading cues to listening in noisy classrooms. A final report of a recent project directed by Frederick Berg, entitled *Listening in Classrooms, Hard of Hearing* (Utah State University, Logan, UT, 1983) includes comprehensive listening data on a group of hard of hearing and near deaf college students. Ralph Belgigue of Comtek has written *Wising Up to Your Companion*. Comparative study of hearing aid and personal FM equipment features is exemplified by an article by David Hawkins in *Journal of Speech and Hearing Disorders* (volume 49, pp. 409–418, 1984). Jerry Jones has recently completed a thesis entitled *Listening of Kindergarten Students Under Close, Distant, and Sound Field FM Amplification Conditions* (Utah State University, Logan, UT 1986).

APPENDIX A

Group 1

1. The (bean) is in the (jar).
2. A (goose) is a large (bird).
3. That yellow (jug) costs a (dime).
4. This (hat) is made from (wood).
5. Please (lock) the (van) doors.
6. The man (dug) a long (ditch).
7. I left my (knife) at (home).
8. I (wish) we had a (kite).
9. Sew the (patch) on my (shirt).
10. Go (pick) a big, (ripe) apple.
11. The (wheel) will (fit) the car.
12. The young (king) was very (mad).
13. The (tooth) is (thin) and white.
14. His (name) is (tough) to spell.
15. A (rose) died in the (Fall).
16. The (sun) warmed the lake (shore).
17. Freddy (sees) a (toad) near him.
18. I (hope) you have a (robe).
19. (Make) a (loop) in your rope.
20. The chicken soup will (boil) (soon).
21. Try to (guess) the correct (route).
22. (Sell) me (that) little, brown dog.
23. (Leave) your (cape) on the bed.
24 Your (mail) is on the (chair).
25 The teacher will (check) each (page).

Group 2

1. Jim will (beg) for a car.
2. The big zooming (jet) is (late).
3. Father will (choose) a car (tire).
4. Put your (coat) on that (rail).
5. I saw mother (burn) the (beef).
6. Fix the (leak) in the (dam).
7. (Dodge) the big, round, (red) ball.
8. Girls (love) to (suck) yellow candy.
9. I (met) Susan at the (gate).
10. (Tall) trees are full of (sap).
11. The (cub) made a lot of (noise).
12. The big (nurse) killed every (germ).
13. Tell me (which) (goal) is ours.
14. I ate (four) pieces of (ham).
15. That green (ring) is a (fake).
16. (Dive) under the water to (hide).
17. (Wash) your dishes in a (pail).
18. (Lead) me to your new (house).
19. The (moon) should (come) up tonight.
20. The big (pan) is too (large).
21. The (pup) will (wag) his tail.
22. Your (chin) moves when you (talk).
23. That (vine) has a long (root).
24. (This) little (seal) loves to swim.
25. The (ship) sailed (south) last night.

Group 3

1. You (did) get my little (note).
2. The (dog) (caught) the blue ball.
3 I (have) a (lame) foot today.
4. I like a big, (cool) (coke).
5. (Shoot) one (young) rabbit for dinner.
6. (Save) the (bun) for the hamburger.
7. Please (pass) me more good (fish).
8. (Join) me for a long (nap).
9. That (sure) was a (dumb) letter.
10. Paint a (mouth) on that (face).
11. I can almost (reach) that (far).
12. The (hill) was a (mile) high.
13. (Geese) are (such) pretty big birds.
14. Stick the (gun) in his (rib).
15. I (bet) you feel very (sad).
16. That man has a (big) (laugh).
17. That tall (pine) tree is (mine).
18. I (lose) money on that (ride).
19. Get that (third) can of (tar).
20. He (led) me to (big) John.
21. The water (hole) (was) very deep.
22. (Jim) went to (vote) last night.
23. (Tap) one (cheek) with your finger.
24. You got my new (tape) (wet).
25. Put the (pearl) in a (sack).

Group 4

1. That is a (nice) (birch) tree.
2. Your (foot) has a broken (bone).
3. The (bug) fell in his (lap).
4. (Shake) the (can) before you pour.
5. We will (give) mother a (wig).
6. (Take) the (date) off the calendar.
7. The (chief) will (hire) three men.
8. The man (said) it would (hail).
9. You can (read) by the (pool).
10. The (path) led to a (mill).
11. (Keep) working on that hard (job).
12. The (lone) ranger (shut) the door.
13. The new (towel) was very (long).
14. Put the (phone) in my (room).
15. (Pack) the (mop) in the car.
16. Catch a (moth) with a (net).
17. The (bus) stopped for some (gas).
18. Spell the (word) "(tool)" for me.
19. Please (serve) the boys some (rice).
20. My (cough) has lasted five (days).
21. Take your (thumb) off that (dish).
22. That is (your) dirty, black (sock).
23. Your (voice) sounds (loud) to me.
24. Please (write) (when) you get home.
25. Go try to (cheer) (him) up.

Group 5

1. Go (bathe) that dirty, old (doll).
2. Lie on your (back) and (sing).
3. Put the (peg) in the (cup).
4. I will (sail) by the (beach).
5. (Tell) me when the (cab) comes.
6. An egg (yolk) can be (food).
7. The (man) fell off the (limb).
8. Take (care) of my new (purse).
9. Get me (five) pieces of (chalk).
10. (Dip) your doughnut in (hot) chocolate.
11. A (town) needs (coal) for heat.
12. Put the (wire) on the (dock).
13. He (let) me wear one (boot).
14. The (judge) wore a (knit) sweater.
15. The paper (match) is (half) burned.
16. Be careful (with) your (sore) foot.
17. With (luck) I'll get some (gum).
18. (Run) and get me a (rock).
19. That green (vase) really looks (good).
20. It is really (mean) to (tease).
21. (Hush) or the (worm) will move.
22. I (need) a long, thin (nail).
23. He (shot) at the lion's (paws).
24. That (light) yellow flower is (real).
26. It rained, (then) the (roof) leaked.

Group 6

1. Go (sit) down, you (bad) boy!
2. I watched the (birth) of a (calf).
3. (Move) that small (tube) of water.
4. I go to (bed) at (night).
5. (Get) a (cage) for the rabbit.
6. (Turn) around and (hit) the ball.
7. The blue (cheese) is all (gone).
8. Put the (chain) on the (door).
9. Jack (paid) me for the (whip).
10. My (niece) played in the (rain).
11. Go (fan) the (fire) a little.
12. Take your (map) on the (hike).
13. Some T.V. (shows) are very (dull).
14. (Search) under the (rug) for money.
15. Tell me one (more) funny (joke).
16. You can (hop) on my (lawn).
17. (Look) at that pretty flower (bud).
18. (Knock) the long, blue (pole) down.
19. The (cat) bit the bird's (wing).
20. All the (team) wore red (shoes).
21. There is a (vowel) in (piece).
22. (Dig) a (well) to find water.
23. (Rush) home and (call) your father.
24. I (live) with my pretty (wife).
25. This (jam) tastes (sour) to me.

Glossary

acoustic: sound, its physical nature.
aided: using a hearing aid.
air–bone gap: decibel difference between air and bone conduction thresholds.
air conduction: sound from the outside air delivered through the ear canal, the eardrum, and the middle ear to the cochlea.
ambient noise: sounds of the environment that are not a part of the desired signal.
absorption: taking in and not reflecting; dissipating in the form of heat.
amplifier: device that increases the intensity of the electrical signal.
analog: continuously variable, e.g., precisely follows sound intensity change.
articulation: vocal tract movements that modify the expired air stream and change the resonating cavities in various ways during the production of consonants and vowels.
assistive listening device: an instrument that enables a person to listen effectively from a distance or in the presence of room noise or room reverberation.
attenuator: a control for reducing the intensity of pure tone or speech signals of an audiometer.
audiology: study of hearing and hearing problems.
audiologist: a nonmedical specialist who studies hearing problems and how to alleviate them.
audiometer: a pure tone instrument for the measurement of sound detection, comfortable loudness range, and uncomfortable loudness level; a speech instrument for the measurement of speech detection and reception thresholds and percentage of speech discrimination or recognition.
audiometric test booth: an enclosure built of dense materials to prevent environmental sounds from keeping faint test stimuli from being heard.

auditory stimulation: delivering sound stimuli to one or more listeners.
auditory-visual stimulation: delivering sound stimuli and accompanying sight stimuli to one or more listeners.
auricle: the outer part of the ear; the pinna.

babble: repetitive or flexible vocal activity of infants before they use meaningful speech.
barrier: a thing that prevents going ahead, as a fence or wall.
basal: forming the base, e.g., the bottom turn of the cochlea.
better ear: ear with better hearing of two impaired ears, determined by sound detection thresholds and sound discrimination or recognition scores.
bilateral: two ears.
binaural: two hearing aids.
bisensory: stimulating the auditory and visual senses simultaneously.
bone conduction: sound delivered to the cochleas by directly vibrating the bone of the skull of a listener with a bone receiver (vibrator).
bone conduction eyeglass: a rare kind of hearing aid in which the amplified electrical signal is transduced via a vibrator into a vibrotactile signal at the left or right mastoid bone.
bone vibrator: a receiver placed against the bone of the head to change an electrical signal into a vibratory signal that is delivered through the skull directly to the cochleas of the ears.
bore: a drilled hole in an earmold through which amplified sound travels.

cassette recorder: a tape recorder and playback unit with a small cartridge of magnetic tape.
chain reaction: a sequence of events, each of which results in or has an effect upon the following event or events.
circuit: an interconnected group of resistors, capacitors, or other internal electronic components.
closed set: a group of items to be discriminated in which the options are known beforehand.
code: a system of symbols for representing information and the rules for associating the symbols.
cochlea: spiral-shaped organ of the inner ear.
cognitive: having to do with cognition, knowing, perceiving, sensing, or being aware.
comfortable listening level: sound that is intense enough to be detected easily but not so intense as to be uncomfortably loud.
complex sound: a sound made up of two or more frequencies.
consonant: a speech sound characterized by constricted voiced or voiceless breath flow through the vocal tract.
consonant blend: a cluster of two or three consonants appearing together at the beginning or at the end of a syllable or word.
cortex: gray matter of the cerebrum of the brain.
cortices: plural of cortex; cortex of each side of the brain.
compression: channeling of a signal into the reduced hearing range of a hearing

impaired person.

compression attack: signal going into compression phase of amplification.

compression release: signal going out of compression phase of amplification.

conductive component: that part of a hearing loss resulting from pathology of the outer ear or middle ear.

corrosion: chemical substance that eats away or destroys material.

conductive mechanism: outer ear, ear canal, eardrum, and middle ear bones.

criteria: a standard for task completion, often expressed in terms of number of correct responses or percentage of correct responses.

crystal: a piece of quartz that vibrates freely at a specific frequency.

decibel (dB): the logarithmic unit of sound intensity or sound pressure.

decode: to translate from an incomprehensible form of information to an understandable form.

demodulate: separate an audio frequency signal from a radio frequency signal.

diaphragm: a vibrating partition that produces sound.

diffraction: the bending or changing of direction of a wave because of striking an edge, a narrow opening, or a new medium.

digital: classifying into numerical categories, usually in sets of two, as opposed to analog, or continuously variable.

direct sound: sound that reaches a location by direct, straight line propagation from the sound source.

directional microphone: a microphone that is more sensitive to sound coming from one direction than from another direction.

distortion: adding or taking away from the original form of a signal.

earhook: extension of behind-the-ear (BTE) hearing aid that conducts amplified sound from the aid to the tubing, which in turn conducts amplified sound to the earmold.

earmold: a cast of the part of the ear where sound enters the ear, which is attached to a hearing aid.

earphone: a receiver within a circular cushion that is worn over an ear and changes an electrical signal into a sound signal.

earshot: the distance over which a person can detect the presence of sound; varies with sound intensity, sound reflection, and hearing sensitivity.

echo: the repeating of a sound produced by sound waves from a surface.

effector: muscle capable of responding to a nerve impulse.

electret microphone: a high fidelity, rugged microphone that is relatively insensitive to structure-borne vibration.

electroacoustic: electronic processing of sound.

electrochemical: production of electricity by chemical changes.

electromagnetic: transduction of sound from an electrical signal to a magnetic signal.

electrotactile: also called vibrotactile; transduces amplified electrical signal into strong tactile or vibrational signal, which stimulates the surface of the body of the user.

environmental microphone: a microphone built in or added to an FM receiver for input of sound from the environment surrounding the listener.

environmental sounds: the myriad of nonspeech sounds such as a doorbell ringing or footsteps.

eustachian tube: a slender canal between the pharynx and the middle ear cavity.

feedback: return of part of the output of a response so as to modify or monitor the response.

formants: concentrations of sound energy into certain frequency bands due to vocal tract resonances; vary from one consonant or vowel to another.

frequency: rate of occurrence of a vibration; the number of times that any regularly repeated event, such as vibration, occurs in a given unit of time.

frequency modulation: modifying the frequency aspect of a radio frequency signal by superimposing an audio frequency signal on it, prior to its being transmitted.

frequency range: lowest to highest frequencies of a signal effectively amplified.

frequency response: relative amplification of each frequency of a signal.

fundamental frequency: the lowest frequency or rate of vibration of a complex sound, or sound with two or more simultaneously occurring vibration rates or frequencies.

gain: amount of amplification in decibels (dB).

gain control: volume control for changing hearing aid amplification in decibels.

genetic: having to do with genes, with origin, and with natural growth.

hair cell: a cochlear cell with very fine hairlike processes.

homeostasis: tendency of an organism to maintain internal equilibrium, notwithstanding external influences.

horn effect: expanding or enlarging the sound bore of an earmold from its entrance to its exit.

immittance: refers to both impedance and admittance.

impedance: total opposition to energy flow.

impedance meter: a device for measuring the impedance or compliance (opposite) of the ear to incoming sound; interchangeably referred to as immittance meter if measuring compliance.

impulse: a surge of electrical current along nerve fibers.

incus: the middle bone of a chain of three small bones in the middle ear.

inflection: pitch change during speech.

integrated circuit: an interconnected group of a great many electronic components in a tiny chip of semiconducting material.

intelligibility: percent of speech understood.

intensity: amount or degree of something, e.g., sound, that can be measured physically.

intonation: pitch change within a syllable or from syllable to syllable in a word, phrase, or sentence.

language: a spoken or written system for communicating thoughts and feelings.

larynx: the structure of muscle and cartilage at the upper end of the windpipe, containing the vocal folds and serving as the organ of voice.
lavalier microphone: a microphone that is attached below the neck of a person.
logarithmic: nonlinear increase or decrease based upon powers of 10.
loudspeaker: a device with a diaphragm that changes an amplified electrical signal into an amplified sound signal that can be heard by many persons simultanously.

magnetic field: space around wire carrying electricity in which magnetic energy exists.
malleus: the outermost of the three small bones of the middle ear.
manner of articulation: the way a consonant sound is produced in distinction to where it is produced; constriction, continuity, and direction of expired air flow during speech.
mask: render a sound signal inaudible with a coexisting competing sound.
mastoid bone: a hard protrusion of the temporal bone directly behind an external ear.
maternal rubella: German measles contracted by mother during the first three months of her pregnancy.
maximum power output: greatest possible intensity of a hearing aid receiver.
meningitis: a dangerous infectious disease in which the membranes surrounding the brain or spinal cord are inflamed.
meter: a unit of length in the metric system equal to 39.37 inches.
microphone: device that changes sound signals into electrical signals.
microphone-telecoil switch: a two-position hearing aid control for changing from microphone input of a sound signal to corresponding telecoil input of the signal.
milliamp: a thousandth of an ampere; a tiny amount of electrical current.
modulate: superimpose an audio frequency signal on a radio frequency signal.
modular: standard or universal, not custom.
molecule: the smallest particle of an element or compound that can exist in free state and still retain the characteristic of the element or compound.
monaural: one hearing aid; aid on one ear.
morphology: pertaining to word stems, prefixes, and suffices, and their meanings.
motor activity: involving muscle movement.

nazalize: produce a speech sound through the nose by opening a back port into the nose.
natural: in speech, refers to utterance that is correct enough to be acceptable to uncritical listeners.
neophrene: synthetic rubber, which is highly resistant to oil, heat, light, and oxidation.
neural: referring to nerves or transmission of impulses through them.
noise: unwanted sound that interferes with communication, is disturbing, or is hazardous to health.

noise cancelling microphone: a transducer that has an inlet to each side of its diaphragm and that is constricted so that ambient noise surrounding it is neutralized and voice input is made very dominant.
noise-lock: treating edges of a door with a magnetic sealing material to prevent air and sound from passing between the door and the door frame.
noise reduction: the intensity in decibels by which sound is reduced from outside to inside a room.
nonreverberant room: an enclosure in which sound reflection is minimal.
normal hearing: standard against which to compare hearing loss; approximately 0 decibels on audiometric scale and 100 percent speech discrimination score or close to it.

occlusion: a blockage of a passageway.
omnidirectional microphone: transducing device that is equally sensitive to sound coming from any direction.
open mold: earmold that permits sound to enter the ear canal without going through the hearing aid.
open set: items to be repeated in which options are unknown beforehand.
oral-nasal distinction: speech sound difference dependent upon whether sound is produced through the mouth or through the nose.
orosensory: referring to sensation in the muscles of the mouth.
ossification: bony growth that replaces elastic tissue between one or more of the middle ear bones; results in hearing loss.
otitis: inflamation of an ear.
otologist: a medical doctor who specializes in the diagnosis and treatment of pathologic conditions of the ear.
otoscope: an instrument for direct examination of the ear canal and eardrum, and indirect examination of the middle ear by its reflection on the eardrum.
output range: fixed minimum to maximum decibel levels of the receiver of the hearing aid when sound entering the aid varies widely in intensity.

partition: something that separates or divides; wall, ceiling, or floor of a room.
pathologic condition: unhealthy condition or process due to disease or other causes.
pediatrician: medical doctor who specializes in children's diseases.
personal FM: a frequency modulation radio system that enables a listener to hear a mobile speaker with minimal noise and reverberation interference.
pharynx: part of vocal tract between larynx and mouth and nose.
phonologic: carryover of speech skills into meaningful words, spoken language, and spoken communication.
place of articulation: vertical and horizontal locations where speech organs come together in and around the mouth.
porous: full of pores or tiny holes enabling sound energy to dissipate in the form of heat.
pragmatic: functional or useful.

prelinguistic: period of life prior to the time children say their first words.
preset: adjust a control of a device before it is used.
programmed: sequence from easy to difficult, to enhance learning.
propagate: extend, project, or travel through space.
proprioceptive: kinesthetic and tactile sensation.
prosodic: stress and intonation features of speech.
public address system: one or more immobile microphones, an amplifier, and one or more loudspeakers used to amplify speech or music and enhance the listening of all people within earshot.
pure tone: sound with one frequency or a single rate of vibration.

radio receiver: device that picks up a transmitted radio signal, demodulates the audio frequency signal from it, amplifies the audio signal, and delivers it to listeners.
radio transmitter: device that modulates the frequency of a radio signal with an audio frequency signal and broadcasts the modulated signal.
real ear sound measurement: determining the physical benefit of a hearing aid and earmold system by comparing amplified and unamplified sound in the ear of the user.
receiver: part of a hearing aid that transduces the amplified electrical signal into an amplified sound signal.
redundancy: part of message that can be eliminated without loss of information.
reflection: directing back of sound or optimal signals by a barrier or partition.
release time: period in which amplified signal is not compressed or limited.
residual hearing: amount of hearing remaining after hearing loss has occurred.
reverberant sound: sound which reaches a given location in a room only after being reflected from one or more barriers or partitions within that room.
reverse slope: audiogram with poorest detection thresholds at low speech frequencies, next poorest at middle speech frequencies, and best detection thresholds at high speech frequencies.
rhythm: recurring pattern of speech or music; in speech, the combination of accent, emphasis, phrasing, intonation, and rate.

schema: diagram, plan, or arrangement.
semantic: meaning of words or word groups.
sensorineural mechanism: cochlear and adjacent part of auditory nerve.
sensory: reception of information through the senses, such as the ears and eyes.
sensory aid: a device that enhances a correct listening or speech response, e.g., a hearing aid or a speech aid.
sensory condition: listening auditorily, visually or through lipreading, or through a combination of audition and vision.
sensory cue: a stimulus that enhances a correct response, e.g., the vibration of the noise during the production of the /m/ sound can be sensed by placing a fingertip against the nose.
sensory stimulation: saying a speech target as many times as needed to assist

children to sense how they should say that target.
servo control: automatic control of a response due to feedback of information from the response.
sign communication: conveying information with hand, arm, and body positions and movements that are arbitrarily given meaning as words and thoughts.
shell: a mold within which an in-the-ear hearing aid is placed or built.
signal: sound that carries information that listeners want to hear.
signal-to-noise ratio: difference between intensity of desired sound in decibels and intensity of competing sound in decibels.
sound: propagated vibration that can be heard.
sound field FM: a frequency modulation radio system with loudspeakers that enables a class of students to listen to a mobile talker.
sound level meter: instrument to measure intensity of sound waves in air, consisting of a microphone, an amplifier, a frequency weighting circuit, and a meter that reads in decibels.
sound transmission loss: logarithmic ratio of the sound intensity in decibels on one side of a partition to the sound intensity in decibels on the other side.
spectrum: a visual display of the separate frequencies of a sound and their individual amplitudes.
speculum: a miniature cone-shaped funnel that is inserted into the ear canal during hearing screening with the acoustic otoscope.
speech discrimination score: percentage of a list of familiar words repeated correctly, or percentage of closed-set word items responded to correction.
speech-language pathologist: a specialist who studies speech and language disorders and how to alleviate them.
stapes: the innermost of the three small bones of the middle ear.
static: electrical discharges in a radio causing noises that interfere with signal reception.
stethoscope: a hearing instrument used to listen to various features of sound through a hearing aid.
stress: accent of syllable or emphasis of word.
suspended: hung by a support from above, e.g., acoustical tile suspended from ceiling.
syllable: one or more connected speech sounds with a vowel nucleus; a basic unit of speech production.
symmetrical: audiograms for both ears having the same configuration.
syntactic: language meaning conveyed from sequence of words in a sentence.

tactile: sense of touch from contact of structures of the mouth, from air constriction in the vocal tract, or from vibration of the vocal folds during speech.
telecoil: a series of interconnected wire loops that respond electrically to a magnetic signal.
terminal: either end of an electrical cord or cable.
threshold: a narrow intensity range where a person is uncertain whether he or she detects the presence of sound.

tone control: knob for adjusting the frequency response of a hearing aid or similar device.
toxin: having to do with or caused by a poison.
transmit: go from one place to another.
trauma: an abnormal physical or mental condition caused by a wound, injury, or shock.
treatment: a condition under which subjects of an experiment are studied.
tubing: plastic hollow material that channels and directs sound in hearing aid systems.
tumor: an abnormal body growth that may be benign or malignant.
tympanum: the middle part of the ear; temporal bone cavity, eardrum, or both.
typanogram: a graph of the mobility of the eardrum while air pressure is varied in the ear canal.

unisensory: stimulating or using one sense at a time during listening.
unoccupied: people not present.
usable gain: that part of the amplification capability of a hearing aid that can benefit a user.

vent: in addition to sound bore, a drilled hole in the earmold of a behind-the-ear hearing aid or in the shell of an in-the-ear hearing aid.
vibrotactile: see electrotactile.
vocal folds: vocal cords; ligaments and supportive tissue of the larynx that may be set into vibration to produce voiced speech sounds.
vocal tract: a passageway from the larynx to the front of the mouth, and sometimes to the front of the nose, which modifies the sound produced by the larynx or within which additional sound is generated during speech.
vocalization: using voice during nonmeaningful utterance or speech.
voice: sound produced by a combination of vibration of the vocal folds and resonance of the vocal tract.
voiced-voiceless distinction: differentiation of two sounds because one is produced with vocal fold vibration and the other without vocal fold vibration.
volume: the length × width × height of a space in cubic units.
vowel: any speech characterized by unconstricted voice flow through the vocal tract.

wall circuit: wire route through which electricity flows in a wall of a room.
warranty: the seller's guarantee to the buyer that the goods are sold as represented and will be replaced and serviced according to the contract between the two parties.
wave form: a graph of a wave showing its amplitude over time.
windscreen: covering placed over a microphone inlet to keep wind noise, breath, and low frequency energy out of a hearing aid or frequency modulation (FM) radio transmitter.
word recognition: identification of a word as evidenced by repeating it when heard.

References

Agnew, J. (1985). In-office analysis of malfunctioning ITE aids. *Hearing Instruments, 36* (10), 20, 22, 24, 26, 28, 76.
American Speech and Hearing Association, Committee on Audiometric Evaluation. (1974). Guidelines for audiometric symbols. *ASHA, 16,* 260–264.
Amon, C. (1981). Meeting state and federal guidelines. In R. Roeser and M. Downs (Eds.), *Auditory disorders in school children* (pp. 18–31). New York: Thieme-Stratton.
Atkinson, R., and Shiffrin, R. (1971). The control of short-term memory. *Scientific American, 225,* 82–90.
Auditory skills instructional planning system. Los Angeles County Schools. North Hollywood: Foreworks.
Belgigue, R. *Wising up to your companion: Instructions for operating your Comtek Companion AT-72.* Salt Lake City: Comtek.
Berg, F. (1976). *Educational audiology: Hearing and speech management.* New York: Grune and Stratton.
Berg, F. (1986). Characteristics of a target population. In F. Berg, J. Blair, S. Viehweg, and A. Wilson-Vlotman (Eds.), *Educational audiology for the hard of hearing child* (pp. 1–24). Orlando, FL: Grune and Stratton.
Berg, F. (1986). Home study phonetics course. Logan, UT: Utah State University.
Berg, F. (1986). *Speech handbook.* Smithfield, UT: Ear Products and Services.
Berg, F., and Child, D. (1986). *Listening refinement program.* Smithfield, UT: Ear Products and Services.
Berg, F., Blair, J., Frantz, J., Ivory, R., Viehweg, S., and Watkins, S. (1983). *Listening in classrooms, hard of hearing.* Final report, Regional Educational Programs for Deaf and Other Handicapped Persons (Postsecondary). Grant No. G008101357, U.S. Department of Education. Logan: Utah State University.

Bergstrom, L. (1981) Medical problems and their management. In R. Roeser and M. Downs (Eds.) *Auditory disorders in school children* (pp. 102–119). New York: Thieme-Stratton.

Bess, F. (1982). Children with unilateral hearing loss. *Journal of Academy of Rehabilitative Audiology, 15,* 131–144.

Birch, J. (1975). *Hearing impaired children in the mainstream.* Reston, VA: Council for Exceptional Children.

Blair, J. (1976). *The contributing influences of amplification, speechreading and classroom environments on the ability of hard of hearing children to discriminate sentences.* Unpublished doctoral dissertation. Northwestern University, Evanston, IL.

Blair, J. (1977). The effects of amplification, speechreading, and classroom environments on reception of speech. *Volta Review, 77* (7), 443–449.

Blair, J., Peterson, M., and Viehweg, S. (1985). The effect of mild hearing loss on academic performance among young school-age children. *Volta Review, 87* (2), 87–94.

Boothroyd, A. (1982). *Hearing impairments in young children.* Englewood Cliffs, NJ: Prentice-Hall.

Boothroyd, A. (1985). Residual hearing and the problem of carry-over in the speech of the deaf. In J. Lauter (Ed.), *Proceedings of the conference on the planning and production of speech in normal and hearing-impaired individuals.* Washington, DC: ASHA Reports 15, pp. 8–14.

Borden, G., and Harris, K. (1984). *Speech science primer.* Baltimore: Williams and Wilkins.

Bowe, C. (1985). Memory issues in speech planning and production. In J. Lauter (Ed.), *Proceedings of the conference on the planning and production of speech in normal and hearing-impaired individuals.* Washington, DC: ASHA Reports 15, pp. 61–69.

Calvert, D. (1980). *Descriptive phonetics.* New York: Thieme-Stratton.

Calvert, D., and Silverman, S. R. (1975). *Speech and deafness. Washington, DC: Alexander Graham Bell Association for the Deaf.*

Clark, T., and Watkins, S. (1985). Programming for hearing impaired individuals through amplification and home intervention. Logan, UT: Utah State University.

Davis, H. (1979). Anatomy and physiology of the auditory system. In H. Davis, and S. R. Silverman (Eds.), *Hearing and deafness* (pp. 46–83). New York: Holt, Rinehart and Winston.

Davis, H. (1979). Abnormal hearing and deafness. In H. Davis, and S. R. Silverman (Eds.), *Hearing and deafness* (pp. 87–146). New York: Holt, Rinehart and Winston.

Davis, J. (Ed.). (1977). *Our forgotten children: Hard of hearing pupils in our schools.* Minneapolis: University of Minnesota Press.

Duhamel, G., and Yoshioka, P. (1985). Subjective listening techniques for assessing hearing aid function. Part 1: Basic listening tests. *Hearing Instruments, 36* (10), 34, 36, 38, 43, 77.

Erber, N. (1982). *Auditory training.* Washington, DC: Alexander Graham Bell Association for the Deaf.

Erber, N. (1985). *Telephone communication and hearing impairment.* San Diego: College-Hill Press.

Finitzo-Hieber, T. (1981). Classroom acoustics. In R. Roeser and M. Downs, *Auditory disorders in school children* (pp. 250–262). New York: Thieme-Stratton.

Finitzo-Hieber, T., and Tillman, T. (1978). Room acoustics effects on monosyllabic word discrimination ability of normal and hearing impaired children. *Journal of Speech and Hearing Research, 21,* 440–458.

Gengel, R. (1971). Acceptable speech-to-noise ratios for aided speech discrimination of the hearing impaired. *Journal of Auditory Research, 11,* 219–221.

Goldstein, J. (1978). Fundamental concepts in sound measurement. In D. Lipscomb (Ed.), *Noise and audiology* (pp. 3–58). Baltimore: University Park Press.

Goodhill, V. (1979). Ear examination. In V. Goodhill (Ed.), *Diseases, deafness, and dizziness* (pp. 88–103). Hagerstown, MD: Harper and Row.

Goodhill, V., and Brockman, S. (1979). Secretory otitis media. In V. Goodhill (Ed.), *Diseases, deafness, and dizziness* (pp. 307–329). Hagerstown, MD: Harper and Row.

Harris, C. (1979). *Handbook of noise control.* New York: McGraw-Hill.

Hawkins, D. (1984). Comparisons of speech recognition in noise by mildly-to-moderately hearing-impaired children using hearing aids and FM systems. *Journal of Speech and Hearing Disorders, 49,* 409–418.

Hirsch, I. (1985) Conference summary. In J. Lauter (Ed.), *Proceedings of the conference on the planning and production of speech in normal and hearing-impaired individuals.* ASHA Reports, 15, pp. 79–80.

Hirschorn, M. (1982). *Noise control reference handbook.* Bronx, NY: Industrial Acoustics.

Hodgson, W. (1980). *Basic audiometric evaluation.* Baltimore: Williams and Wilkins.

Jerger, J. (1970). Clinical experience with impedance audiometry. *Archives of Otolaryngology, 92,* 311–324.

Johnsson, L., and Hawkins, J. (1976). Degeneration patterns in human ears exposed to noise. *Transactions of the American Otolaryngological Society, 64,* 52–66.

Jones, J. (1966). *Listening of kindergarten students under close, distant, and sound field FM amplification conditions.* Unpublished educational specialist thesis, Utah State University.

Kent, R. (1985). Developing and disordered speech: Strategies for organization. In J. Lauter (Ed.), *Proceedings of the conference on the planning and production of speech in normal and hearing-impaired individuals.* ASHA Reports, 15, pp. 29–37.

Kweskin, S. (1981). *Hearing aids: A guide to their use and wear.* Patient Information Library. Daly City, CA: Krames Communications.

Ladefoged, P. (1967). *Elements of acoustic phonetics.* Chicago: University of Chicago Press.

Lauter, J. (1985). Respiratory function in speech production by normally-hearing and hearing-impaired talkers: A review. In J. Lauter (Ed.), *Proceedings of the conference on the planning and production of speech in normal and hearing-impaired individuals.* ASHA Reports, 15, pp. 58–60.

Leggett, S., Brubaker, C., Cohodes, A., and Shapiro, A. (Eds.). (1977). *Planning flexible learning places.* New York: McGraw-Hill.

Ling, D. (1976). *Speech and the hearing-impaired child.* Washington, DC: Alexander Graham Bell Association for the Deaf.

Ling, D. (1981). *The detection factor* [videotape]. Montreal: McGill University.

Ling, D., and Ling, A. (1978). *Aural habilitation.* Washington, DC: Alexander Graham Bell Association for the Deaf.

MacNeilage, P., Studdert-Kennedy, M., and Lindblom, B. (1985). Planning and production of speech: An overview. In J. Lauter (Ed.), *Proceedings of the conference on the planning and production of speech in normal and hearing-impaired individuals.* ASHA Reports, 15, pp. 15-21.
Martin, F. (Ed.). (1981). *Medical audiology.* Englewood Cliffs: Prentice-Hall.
Musket, C. (1981). Maintenance of personal hearing aids. In R. Roeser and M. Downs (Eds.), *Auditory disorders in school children* (pp. 229-249). New York: Thieme-Stratton.
Nabelek, A., and Nabelek, I. (1978). Principles of noise control. In D. Lipscomb (Ed.), *Noise and audiology* (pp. 59-79). Baltimore: University Park Press.
Nabelek, A., and Nabelek, I. (1985). Room acoustics and speech perception. In J. Katz (Ed.), *Handbook of clinical audiology* (pp. 834-846). Baltimore: Williams and Wilkins.
Nober, L. (1981). Developing IEP's for hard of hearing children. In M. Ross and L. Nober (Eds.), *Special education in transition: Educating hard of hearing children.* Washington, DC: Alexander Graham Bell Association for the Deaf.
Pickett, J. (1980). *The sounds of speech communication: A primer of acoustic phonetics and speech perception.* Baltimore: University Park Press.
Pollack, D. (1985). *Educational audiology for the infant and preschooler.* Springfield, IL: Charles C. Thomas.
Pollack, M. (Ed.). (1980). *Amplification for the hearing-impaired.* New York: Grune & Stratton.
Potter, R., Kopp, H. (1966). *Visible speech.* New York: Dover.
Quigley, S., and Thomure, F. (1968). *Some effects of hearing impairment upon school performance.* Springfield, IL: Division of Special Education Services.
Roeser, R., and Price, D. (1981). Audiometric and impedance measures: Principles and interpretation. In R. Roeser and M. Downs (Eds.), *Auditory disorders in school children* (pp. 71-101). New York: Thieme-Stratton.
Ross, M. (1982). *Hard of hearing children in regular schools.* Englewood Cliffs, NJ: Prentice-Hall.
Sarff, L., Ray, H., and Bagwell, A. (1981). Why not amplification in every classroom? *Hearing Aid Journal, 11,* 44, 47-48, 50, 52.
Silverstone, D. M. (1982). Considerations for listening and noise distraction. In P. J. Sleeman and D. Rockwell (Eds.), *Designing learning environments* (p. 79). New York: Longman.
Simon, C. (1980). *Communicative competence: A functional-pragmatic language program.* Tucson: Communication Skills Builders.
Staab, W. (1985). Contemporary practices and trends in hearing aid techniques. [workshop]. Logan: Utah State University, July 25-26.
Stelmach, G., and Hughes, B. (1985). Attention, motor control, and automaticity. In J. Lauter (Ed.), *Proceedings of the conference on the planning and production of speech in normal and hearing-impaired individuals.* ASHA Reports, 15, pp. 22-28.
Stevens, K. (1981). Speech production and acoustic goals. In J. Lauter (Ed.), *Proceedings of the conference on the planning and production of speech in normal and hearing-impaired individuals.* ASHA Reports, 15, pp. 38-42.
Stevens, S., and Davis, H. (1938). *Hearing: Its psychology and physiology.* New York: John Wiley.
Stoker, R., and Spears, J. (1984). Hearing-impaired perspectives on living in the

mainstream [monograph]. *Volta Review, 86,* 5.
Studebaker, G., and Bess, F. (Eds.). (1982). *The Vanderbilt hearing aid report.* Upper Darby, PA: Monographs in Contemporary Audiology.
Viehweg, S. (1986). Audiological considerations. In F. Berg, J. Blair, S. Viehweg, and A. Wilson-Vlotman (Eds.), *Educational audiology for the hard of hearing child* (pp. 81–99). Orlando, FL: Grune and Stratton.
Viehweg, S. (1986). Hearing aids. In F. Berg, J. Blair, S. Viehweg, and A. Wilson-Vlotman (Eds.), *Educational audiology for the hard of hearing child* (pp. 101–130). Orlando, FL: Grune and Stratton.
Warren, D. (1976). Aerodynamics of speech production. In N. Less (Ed.), *Contemporary issues in experimental phonetics* (pp. 105–137). New York: Academic Press.
Wedenberg, E. (1954). Auditory training of severely hard of hearing pre-school children. *Acta Otolaryngologica* (Suppl. 54), 1–29.
Wedenberg, E., and Wedenberg, M. (1970). The advantage of auditory training: A case report. In F. Berg and S. Fletcher (Eds.), *The hard of hearing child* (pp. 319–330). New York: Grune and Stratton.
Wilson-Vlotman, A. (1986). Management and coordination of services to the hard of hearing child. In F. Berg, J. Blair, S. Viehweg, and A. Wilson-Vlotman (Eds.), *Educational audiology for the hard of hearing child* (pp. 181–203). Orlando, FL: Grune and Stratton.

Subject Index

A

Acoustic otoscope
 description, 34–37
 operation, 34–36
 readings, 34–37
 value, 34, 36
Acoustical control plan, 113
Acoustical engineer, 89–90, 113
Acoustical noise; *see also* Reducing noise
 effect on voice, 1
 definition
 floor, 95–96
 levels, 2, 90, 107, 110, 159
 measurement, 98–102
 occupied classroom, 95
 optimal, 98
 sources, 89–90, 107–110, 112–113
 unoccupied, 95
Acoustical treatment
 carpet, 105
 ceiling tile, 105
 doors, 114–116
 fiberglass panels, 105

frequency effect, 105–106
ventilation silencer, 114–115
windows, 114–116
Audiogram
 aided, 119, 124–125
 description, 69
 interpreting, 69
 purpose, 69
 samples, 85–87
 symbols, 69, 84–86
 unaided, 119, 125
Audiologist; *see also* Educational audiologist
 definition, 27
 instruments used by, 28–37, 46, 48, 68–69, 72, 81, 98–102, 131–132, 140–141, 148, 150–152
 understanding, 28
Audiologist, roles of
 classroom acoustics, 90, 113
 evaluating and maintaining FM equipment, 187
 fitting hearing aids, 118, 139
 hearing conservation, 27, 63, 72, 78
 listening testing and training, 78

Audiologist, roles of *(continued)*
  managing hearing aids, 139–152
  overall, 27, 139
  taking ear impressions, 131
Audiometer
  controls, 69
  earphones, 69, 84
  pure tones, 68
  purpose, 68
  vibrator, 83–84
Audiometric room, 114–118
Audioscope, 72, 74
Audition, 65
Auditory processing difficulty, 2

B

Battery
  charger, 179–180, 184
  function, 119
  life, 146–148, 183–184
  types, 146–148, 183

C

Case studies
  FM equipment, 155–156
  hearing aids, 117–118
  hearing considerations, 17–18
  listening considerations, 63–64
  room acoustics, 89–90
  speech considerations, 39–40
Cholesteatoma, 25, 27
Classroom acoustics; *see* Room acoustics
Classroom listening data
  noise effect, 97–98
  normal versus hard of hearing, 97–98
  reverberation effect, 97–98
Classroom teacher, roles of
  FM equipment, 9, 156, 177–187, 189–190
  hearing aids, 8–9, 118, 142–153
  hearing problems, 6, 7–8, 30–34, 36, 37–38
  listening problems, 7, 64, 67, 69, 72, 75, 77–81
  room acoustics, 7–8, 90, 102–103, 105, 107, 109, 113
  speech problems, 7, 40, 42, 43, 46, 48, 49, 52, 61
Classroom teachers
  number in United States, 5
  professional preparation, 5–6
  training needed, 5–9

D

Decibels, 27, 68–76, 82, 85–86, 89, 93–102, 107, 109–111, 116, 122–126, 159, 161
Discrimination problem, 64
Down's syndrome
  description, 24
  hearing loss, 24
Duration of speech syllables, 41

E

Ear
  parts of, 20–21
  wax, 27, 31
Earmolds; *see also* Shells
  damping elements, 128, 130
  definition, 193
  horn effect, 128, 130
  materials, 131
  reconfigure sound, 119, 130
  types, 131, 133
  vents, 128, 130
Educational audiologists
  job task, 3
  need for and number employed, 3
Educational Audiology Association, 15
Educational study room, 116

F

Five sound test, 75, 77, 187
FM equipment; *see also* Personal FM equipment, Sound field FM equipment
  audiovisual options, 165, 180–181
  basic components, 158, 164–168
  benefits, 158
  sound field versus personal, 157–158, 161
FM equipment evaluation and maintenance
  companies, 186
  criteria, 186
  description, 186
  five sound test, 187
  minor servicing, 186
  sentence lists, 187, 189–190
  user precautions, 186
FM microphone
  directional versus nondirectional, 164–166
  hand-held versus wearable, 165–166
  lavalier style, 165–166
  noise cancelling, 165–166
  price, 165
  self-contained directional, 165–166
  windscreen, 165
FM receiver
  crystal modules, 169–171
  hearing aid option, 169, 173
  personal and sound field options, 168–170
  subcomponents, 168
  wearable options, 170
FM signals
  "live," 165
  radio frequencies, 168
  recorded and broadcast, 165–168
FM transmitter
  carrying pouches, 168
  input options, 167–168, 182–183
  operations, 168
  wearable options, 168–169

Foreign bodies in ear canal, 31
Frequency of sound, 83
Frequency modulation (FM)
  broadcast band, 157
  compared with amplitude modulation (AM), 157
  components, 158, 164–177
  process, 157

H

Hard of hearing; *see also* Hearing loss, Listening deficit
  educational deficit, 13–15, 39, 117
  identification, 12–13, 71–72
  language deficit, 13–15, 58–59
  listening problems, 2–3, 64, 70–71, 78, 81
  secondary consequences, 1, 39, 117
  versus normal hearing and deaf, 1, 12–13, 42
Hearing
  comparison with vision, 18–19
  functions, 18–19
  language, thought, and speech, 19
  sound, 18
Hearing aid; *see also* Hearing aid features
  benefit, 40, 64, 89, 118, 156
  binaural, 118–119, 155
  candidates, 122–124
  description, 118–119, 139
  fitting required, 118, 131–133
  in noise and reverberation, 2
  monaural, 118
  noise suppressor, 89
  source materials, 153–154
Hearing aid components; *see also* Battery
  amplifier, 118–120, 124–125, 133
  earhook, 122
  microphone, 119, 133

Hearing aid components
(continued)
  speaker or receiver, 120, 131
  telecoil, 136-137
  tubing, 122
Hearing aid controls
  battery compartment, 133
  compression, 126-127, 133
  gain or volume, 119, 124-125, 133
  output, 127-128
  screwdriver, 121, 133
  switches, 133, 136-138
  tone, 127-130, 133
Hearing aid features; see also Battery, Earmolds, Hearing aid components, Hearing aid controls
  acoustic feedback, 125
  adaptive compression, 138-139
  amplification or gain, 118-120, 124-125
  compression, 119, 126-127, 138-139
  frequency adjustments, 127-130
  noise control, 137-139
  output, 127-128
  reconfiguration, 118
  transduction, 119-120, 131
Hearing aid fittings
  binaural versus monaural, 118, 131-133
  unilateral, 131-133
Hearing aid management program
  description, 139-154
  moisture control, 143-146
  performance checks, 140
  servicing, 140-154
  team of persons, 139-140
  visual checks, 142-149
  warranties, 140
Hearing aid management, equipment and supplies
  battery tester, 148
  cleaning materials, 142-146
  current drain meter, 140
  moisture control, 143-146
  stethoscope, adaptor, and connecting tube, 150
  test boxes, 140-141
Hearing aid problems
  batteries, 146-149
  disconnection of parts, 148-149
  moisture, 143-146
  sound stoppage, 148-149
  squeal, 149-150
Hearing aid styles or types
  behind-the-ear (BTE), 120-121
  body, 120-121
  contralateral routing of signals (CROS), 131-133
  eyeglass, 120-122
  in-the-ear (ITE), 120-122
Hearing conservation
  antihistamines and anticongestants, 31
  audiological assistance, 27-28
  considerations, 27
  medical care, 25-26
Hearing loss; see also Hard of hearing, Listening deficit
  average, 69, 117
  bilateral, 42, 57, 70
  conditions and causes, 22-25, 63
  conductive, 22, 39, 70, 127
  degree, 1, 69; see also Audiograms
  description, 22
  mixed, 22
  physical symptoms and behaviors, 37-38
  prevalence, 1
  test for experiencing, 1
  unilateral, 1, 69, 131-135
Hearing screening
  candidates, 72
  instruments used, 72
  procedures, 72
Hearing tests; see also Audiometer
  air conduction, 83-87
  bone conduction, 83-87
  masking, 86
  procedure, 68, 83, 86
  purpose, 67
  stimuli, 67
How we hear, 21-22

Subject Index 211

I

Individualized educational programs (IEPS); *see also* Public Law 94-142
  area of need, 64
  classroom teacher roles, 12
  content, 11
  hearing aid management, 139-140
  number written for hearing impaired, 11
  student study team, 11-12, 64
Impedance meter; *see also* Tympanogram
  description, 31-32
  function, 31
  types, 31
  value, 32
Instruments to identify hearing loss
  acoustic otoscope, 34-36
  audiometer, 68, 72
  audioscope, 72
  impedance meter, 31-34
  otoscope, 28-31
  pneumatic otoscope, 29
Intensity; *see* Sound intensity
International Phonetic Alphabet (IPA), 43-44

L

Language
  development of, 19
  reading and writing, 19
Language training; *see also* Simon program
  deaf versus hard of hearing, 66-67
  early, 66
Listening
  definition, 65
  importance, 65
  role in school, 3
  time in school, 3
  value for language, 3
Listening attitude, 66

Listening development,
  description, 66
  stimulation and training in, 66
Listening deficit; *see* Hard of hearing, Hearing loss
Listening performance, 64
Listening problems, 71-72, 90
Listening program; *see* Listening training
Listening range, 71
Listening training
  benefits, 67
  deaf versus hard of hearing, 66-67
  objective, 78
  school curricula, 67
  self-instruction, 80-81
  sensory precedence, 78
  source materials, 81-82
  stages, 67
  tasks, 66, 78-80
  test, 77-78
  tutoring, 66
Loudness of voice, 41

M

Message-to-competition ratio; *see* Signal-to-noise ratio

N

Noise; *see* Acoustic noise

O

Open plan classrooms, 112
Otitis media
  acute, 30-31
  chronic, 22, 31
  definition, 22
  hearing loss, 22
  recurrent, 18, 22, 31
  serous, 18, 22, 29, 31

Otological care, 26–27
Otologist; *see also* Otological care
  possible treatments, 27
  role in hearing conservation, 25, 63
Otoscope; *see also* Instruments to identify hearing loss
  caution in using, 30
  description, 28
  function, 28
  screening value, 30
  simple versus pneumatic, 29

P

Pathologic conditions of ear
  diagnosis, 31
  possible, 29, 31
Pediatrician, 25
Personal FM benefits
  earshot 158, 182
  signal-to-noise ratio, 161, 163
  signal intensity, 125–126
  speech recognition, 156, 161, 163
Personal FM equipment
  candidates, 161–164
  components, 156, 158
Personal FM operation
  batteries, 183
  battery charger, 184
  covers, 185
  crystal, 184–185
  direct input, 181–183
  magnetic input, 181–183
  receiver unit, 179, 181–182, 184
  recording speech, 180–181
  switch and lights, 185
  transmitter unit, 177, 181
  transmitting recorded stimuli, 180–182
Phonetics course, 52
Pitch of voice, 41, 50–51
Preferential seating, 114

Public health nurse
  number in schools, 28
  role in hearing conservation, 25–26, 28
Public Law 94–142
  provisions, 28
  relation to hearing loss, 28

R

Reducing noise; *see also* Sound transmission losses
  air-borne sound, 109–112
  child-generated, 109
  policies, 107
  structure-borne sound, 107, 109–110, 112
  wall barriers, 107–112, 114–116
Regular and special educators; *see also* Classroom teachers
  special training in listening management for, 5–9
  traditional professional preparation, 5
Regular teachers; *see* Classroom teachers
Reverberation; *see* Room reverberation, Reverberation time
Reverberation time; *see also* Sound absorption coefficients
  description, 105
  formula for estimation, 102–103
  minimally acceptable, 97
  optimal, 98
Room acoustics, 89–116
  factors, 90–91
  listening problem, 2, 91
  maintenance, 90
  measurement, 90
  noise levels, 2, 90
  noise sources, 89–90
  reverberation, 2, 91–93
  source materials, 114

Subject Index

study committee, 90
treatment, 90
Room reverberation; *see also*
  Reverberation time
  alleviation, 103, 105
  description, 91–92
  smearing effect, 91–92
  time, 93, 97–98

S

School nurse; *see* Public health nurse
Shells; *see also* Earmolds
  function, 12
  frequency modifications, 128, 130
  materials, 131
  types, 131
Signal, 65; *see also* Signal-to-noise ratio
Signal-to-noise ratio, 95, 97–98, 109, 133–135, 163–164
Simon program
  application, 61
  description, 59–61
  supplementary material, 61
Simulating hearing loss, 72–73, 75–76
Sound absorption coefficients, 103–104
Sound field FM benefits
  academic achievement, 159–160
  class attention and participation, 156, 178
  cost, 160–161
  earshot, 158
  signal intensity, 125–126
  signal-to-noise ratio, 161
  teacher mobility, 159, 161, 163
  voice protection, 156
Sound field FM equipment
  battery options, 177
  candidates, 159–161
  components, 158, 164–168, 178
  operation; *see* FM operation
  use, 156, 158–159
Sound intensity, 82, 87, 125–126
Sound localization, 66
Sound propagation, 91
Sound transmission losses, 109–111
Speech
  breathing, 55
  feedback, 54–55
  goals or "targets," 56
  hierarchy, 53
  meaningful, 53
  memory role, 53–54
  nonmeaningful, 53
  phonation cycle, 55–56
  phonemic features, 53
  planning and production, 53
  preplanning, 54
  rate, 54
  redundant features, 56
  understandable, 56
Speech aid; *see* Vocal scope
Speech aspects
  articulation, 51
  breath, 50
  intensity, 56
  intonation, 51
  nasality, 51
  pitch, 50, 56
  stress, 50
  voice, 50
Speech check
  description, 49
  procedure, 49
Speech comprehension, 65
Speech cues
  deep, 57
  surface, 56
Speech detection, 65, 67
Speech development
  bilateral versus unilateral hearing loss, 42, 57–58
  levels and skills, 58
  normal sequence, 42
  parent and teacher role, 42

Speech discrimination, 65
Speech mechanism parts, 40–41
Speech perception
  residual hearing versus lipreading cues, 57
  testing and training, 57
  vocal tract features, 57
Speech power, 75
Speech problem, 50
Speech programs
  description, 46
  index, 45
  number, 45–46
Speech recognition, 65, 70–71, 97–98, 163–164
Speech screening, 49
Speech sounds; *see also* International Phonetic Alphabet
  compared to alphabet letters, 43–45
  in context, 43–44
  incorrect production, 43
  learning to identify, 43
  list, 44
  number, 43
Speech training
  age to begin, 49, 66
  deaf compared with hard of hearing, 52, 66–67
  developmental, 52, 58
  prior evaluation, 52
  programs, 52
  reasons to begin early, 42–43
  resistance from parents, 49
  source materials, 52–53
  tasks, 66
  teamwork, 52
  tutoring, 66
Speech understanding, 70–71, 75

T

Teachers of the hearing impaired
  listening, language, speech training role, 48, 52, 59, 78
  hearing management skills, 5
  methods used by, 4
  responsibility with hearing impaired, 4
Tubes
  artificial, 17
  eustachian, 17
Tympanogram; *see also* Impedance meter
  description, 31–32
  types, 32–33
  value, 32, 34

V

Vision, 65
Vocal scope
  applicable contexts, 48
  applicable sounds, 48
  operation, 46, 48
  patterns, 46, 48
  value, 48